Dedication

To my grandparents . . . *You've built a strong, close, and admirable family—a rarity by today's standards. Our tree stands tall because of the roots held by you both. You demonstrated the meaning of hard work, good times, and the love that can be given only by a grandparent.*

"Nothing is so strong as gentleness, and nothing is so gentle as real strength."—Anonymous

Contents

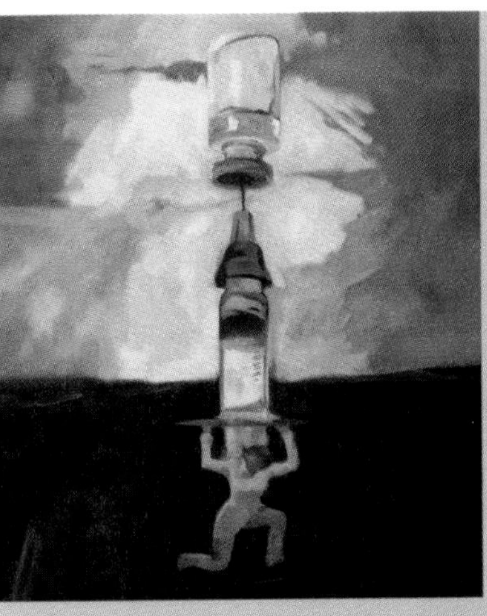

The Pharmacy Technician Series

The Pharmacy Technician Series

The Pharmacy Technician Series

The Pharmacy Technician Series

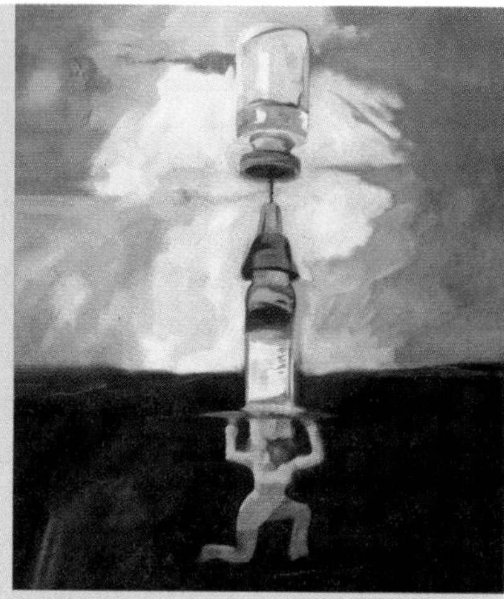

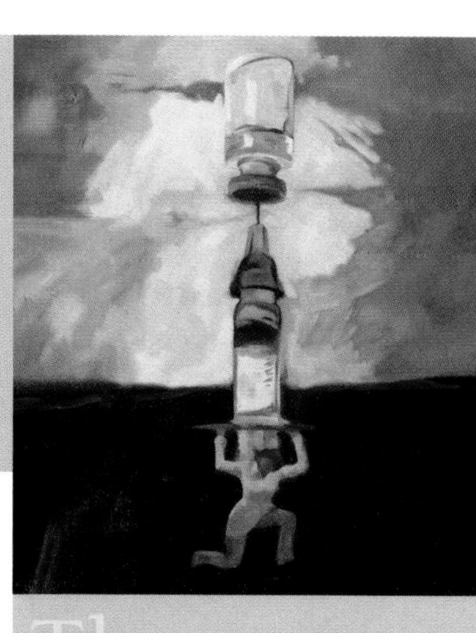

The Pharmacy Technician Series

The Pharmacy Technician Series
The Pharmacy Technician Series
The Pharmacy Technician Series

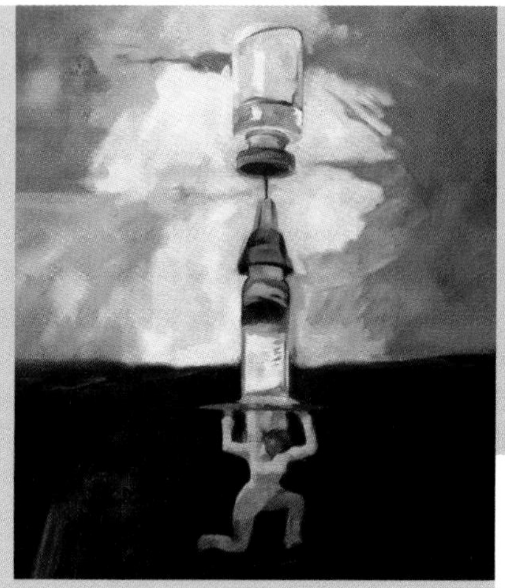

The Pharmacy Technician Series

The Pharmacy Technician Series

The Pharmacy Technician Series

The Pharmacy Technician Series

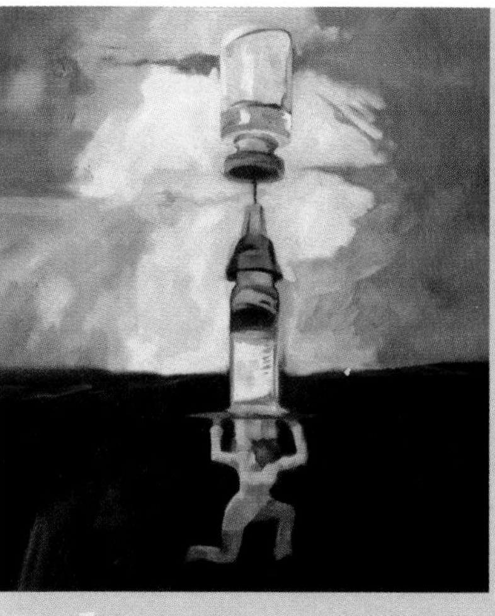

The Pharmacy Technician Series

The Pharmacy Technician Series

The Pharmacy Technician Series

The Pharmacy Technician Series

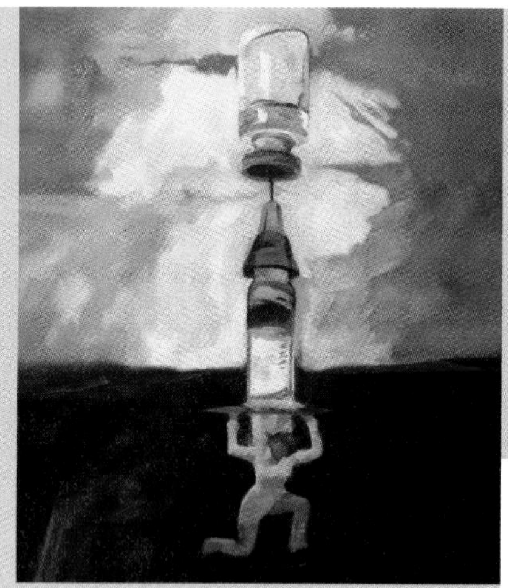

The Pharmacy Technician Series

The Pharmacy Technician Series

The Pharmacy Technician Series

The Pharmacy Technician Series

Preface

Sterile Products is a core title in Prentice Hall's newest series for pharmacy technician education. *The Pharmacy Technician Series* comprises six books that have been developed and designed together, ensuring greater success for the pharmacy technician student.

About the Book

Sterile product preparation and aseptic technique are advanced skills for pharmacy technicians. While this training provides extended career opportunities, it is a challenging and precise skill to learn. This book, however, has been designed to guide the student through with ease, as each theory builds on those presented in earlier chapters.

The core features of this book include the following:

- Chapter introductions and summaries, which provide the student with a clearer understanding and rationale of the content being covered.
- Current, step-by-step instructions with color photographs of various aseptic techniques.
- Workplace Wisdoms provide quick, highlighted tips and comments that replicate the advice of a seasoned IV technician.
- Profiles in Practice provide practical exercises that simulate real-world pharmacy problems or give students the additional information and resources.
- Chapter reviews questions provide a learning assessment for both students and instructors to assess concept comprehension.
- Appendix B, "Common Intravenous Medications," provides a current listing of common IV medications used in the United States. Drugs are categorized alphabetically by both generic name and trade name their use/classification is also provided.
- Appendix C, "Training and Validation Forms," provides documentation that students and instructors can use with lab practicums, skills analysis or, even certification programs.

- Appendix D, "Instructions for Left-Handed Personnel," provides tremendous value for those are left-handed or train individuals who are. Left-handed trainees have been frustrated trying to master aseptic technique for years, as all instructional material has been designed for a right-handed perspective. Step-by-step photos showing left-handed procedures have been included for all baseline aseptic techniques.

About the Series

While a variety of textbooks and training manuals have been available for pharmacy technician education, none met the true educational needs of the industry—until now.

We set out to develop the most comprehensive, accurate, and current texts ever published for pharmacy technicians. One method we used to achieve this goal was involving pharmacy technician educators and trainers from across the country in every phase of the project. You will find that each title in this series has been developed, written, and reviewed exclusively by practicing pharmacy technician educators and practicing pharmacy professionals—a winning approach.

About the Authors

Robin Luke, CPhT

Robin is a founding member of NPTA's Executive Advisory Board—the elected body of leaders for the National Pharmacy Technician Association. She has more than ten years of experience in institutional pharmacy, sterile product preparation, compounding, bulk manufacturing, and management, with a specialized knowledge of herbals and homeopathic treatments.

Robin has developed a variety of continuing-education programs with a strong emphasis on reducing medication errors; she also speaks at meetings and conferences across the United States.

with

Mike Johnston, CPhT

Mike is known internationally as a respected author and speaker in the field of pharmacy. He published his first book, *Rx for Success—A Career Enhancement Guide for Pharmacy Technicians*, in 2002.

In 1999, Mike founded NPTA in Houston, Texas, and led the association from three members to more than 20,000 in less than two years. Today, as executive director of the National Pharmacy Technician Association and publisher of *Today's Technician* magazine, he spends the majority of his time meeting with and speaking to employers, manufacturers, association leaders, and elected officials on issues related to pharmacy technicians.

About NPTA

NPTA, the National Pharmacy Technician Association, is the world's largest professional organization established specifically for pharmacy technicians. The association is dedicated to advancing the value of pharmacy technicians and the vital roles they play in pharmaceutical care. In a society of countless associations, we believe it takes much more than a mission statement to meet the professional needs and provide the needed leadership for the pharmacy technician profession—it takes action and results.

The organization is composed of pharmacy technicians practicing in a variety of practice settings, such as retail, independent, hospital, mail-order, home care, long-term care, nuclear, military, correctional facility, formal education, training, management, and sales. NPTA is a reflection of this diverse profession and provides unparalleled support and resources to members.

NPTA is the foundation of the pharmacy technician profession; we have an unprecedented past, a strong presence, and a promising future. We are dedicated to improving our profession while remaining focused on our members.

For more information on NPTA:
Call 888-247-8700
Visit www.pharmacytechnician.org

Acknowledgments

This book, which is part of a six-title series, has been both an exhilarating and an exhausting project. To say that this series is the result of a collaborative team effort would be a gross understatement.

Special thanks to SaveWay Compounding Pharmacy (Bear, Delaware), PCCA (Professional Compounding Centers of America, Houston, Texas), and Clarian Health System (Indianapolis, Indiana) for your assistance with this text. Nearly every photograph presented throughout this book was shot on location at your facilites. We are grateful for the assistance, patience, and collaboration of your entire staff.

We would also like to thank Jeremy Van Pelt (Photographer) and Multi Med Media (Production Management).

Mark — thank you for believing in my initial vision and concept for this series, which was anything but traditional. I will always remember the day we spent in New York City talking about cover concepts and the like at coffee shops and art galleries. More important, I am honored to have gotten to know you, Alex, and now little Sophie—and I consider each of you friends.

Joan — you are truly gifted at what you do. I am amazed at your ability to join this project at the point you did and to guide each daunting task into a smooth and successful accomplishment. I feel that your leadership has created a better final product.

Julie — thank you for taking risks (plural) on this project, compared with standard policies and procedures. In the end, your support and belief in this project has allowed a truly innovative product to be published.

Robin — your commitment to this project, to exceeding all expectations, and to developing the best training series for pharmacy technicians available has been amazing. You are a wonderful, gifted individual—but most important I am thankful to call you a friend.

Andrew and Jenny — thank you supporting this project, each in your own unique ways; thank you for supporting me and the entire organization. This project tested each of us, our character, and our will, and I am honored to know you both.

Most important, I wish to thank my family. The past several years have been difficult and trying, but the strength, love, and support that you've given me have always pulled me through. ***Thank you***.

Contributors

Jennifer Fix, RPh, MBA
Haltom City, TX

Linda F. McElhiney, Pharm.D., RPh
Clarian Health
Indianapolis, IN

Karen Orth, CPhT
Austin Community College
Austin, TX

Carol Reyes, CPhT
Oncology Specialists, S.C.
Franklin Park, IL

Reviewers

The reviewers of The Pharmacy Technician Series have provided many excellent suggestions and ideas for improving these texts. The quality of the reviews has been outstanding, and the reviews have been a major aid in the preparation of the manuscript. The assistance provided by these experts is deeply appreciated.

Lisa C. Barnes, B. Pharm., MBA
ACPE Program Administrator,
Adjunct Assistant Professor
of Pharmacy Practice
University of Montana School of Pharmacy and Allied Health Sciences
Missoula, Montana

Kimberly Brown, CPhT
Associate Director and Instructor
of Pharmacy Technology
Walters State Community College
Morristown, Tennessee

Ralph P. Casas, Pharm. D., Ph.D.
Associate Professor of Pharmacology
Cerritos Community College
Norwalk, California

Kristie Fitzgerald, BS, Pharm.
Clinical Pharmacist, Department
of Neonatology; Instructor
Salt Lake Community College
Salt Lake City, Utah

Madeline Jensen-Grauel, BS, Ed., M.Sc
Director, Pharmacy Technician Training Program
The University of Texas Medical Branch at Galveston
Galveston, Texas

Robert D. Kwiatkowski, BS, MA
Adjunct Instructor
PIMA Medical Institute
Colorado Springs, Colorado

Herminio Maldonado, Jr., MS, BS
Pharmacy Technician Instructor
PIMA Medical Institute
Colorado Springs, Colorado

Bradley Moore, MSN
Director of Health Science
Remington Administrative Services, Inc.
Little Rock, Arkansas

Hieu Nguyen, BS, CPh.T.
Pharmacy Technician Program Director
Western Career College
Sacramento, California

CHAPTER 1

Introduction to Sterile Products

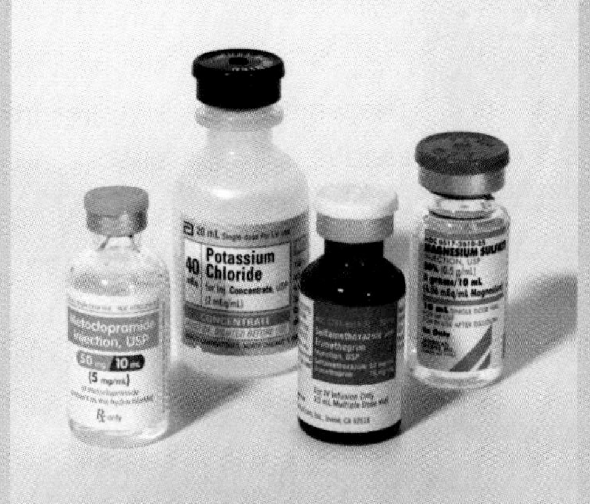

Learning Objectives

After completing this chapter, you should be able to:

- Define aseptic compounding and explain the need for sterile products.
- Distinguish between inhalants, enterals, topicals, ophthalmics, otics, and parenterals as dosage forms used in sterile products.
- Explain why it is important that the parenteral administration route must be sterile or prepared aseptically.
- Distinguish and explain the different forms of parenteral administration.
- Determine which types of parenteral administration must be preservative-free.

INTRODUCTION

Pharmacists and apothecaries have been compounding medications since the first use of medicine. Originally, pharmacists needed to compound most medications from a selection of ingredients, sort of like a recipe. A prescriber would write which active ingredient(s) he wanted the patient to have to treat a certain condition, and the pharmacist, in a chemist-type role, would mix these ingredients together in a base.

The medications we see today that are already prepared, such as tablets, were not always available. It is no longer necessary for the average pharmacy to compound numerous medications. Today we see readily available preparations: syrups, suspensions, ointments, creams, injectables, and many more. However, compounding is still being performed and is still necessary for many other reasons, such as alternative dosing or delivery methods. There are basically two types of compounding. *Extemporaneous compounding* is the nonsterile compounding of oral and topical medications; *aseptic*, or *sterile, compounding* generally refers to IV admixture. Aseptic compounding is the preparation of sterile products intended for a specific route of administration: intravenous, intrathecal, ophthalmic, and many others.

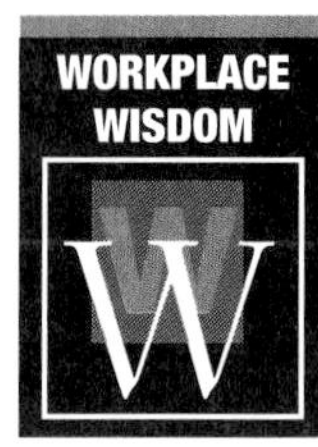

The word *aseptic* comes from the Latin word *a*, meaning "without," and the Latin word *sepsis*, meaning "infection." When using the term *aseptic*, we are talking about making or compounding a product without infection, also referred to as sterile.

pyrogen
a substance that produces fever

Today, technicians generally perform the majority of the actual compounding procedures for sterile products in institutional settings. Pharmacists, however, are still held responsible, legally and ethically, for compounding and dispensing practices in their pharmacies. Pharmacists must be knowledgeable and well qualified in their compounding abilities in order to properly supervise technicians and perform the final check on completed work.

Aseptic technique, as previously discussed, refers to keeping a product sterile. It also refers to different products requiring various manipulations. Still, sterility is always the focus and the pharmacy technician who compounds following all established guidelines is known as someone who practices proper aseptic technique.

The products used in aseptic compounding are manufactured to be sterile, so the IV technician's job is not to introduce any additional **pyrogens**, or fever-causing substances, such as bacteria, fungi, and viruses. Aseptic compounding is accomplished by following a series of specific steps involving aseptic hand-washing procedures, wearing proper and protective dress, knowledge and skill regarding equipment such as the laminar air-flow hood, and solid product manipulation skills.

Routes of Administration

There are numerous routes of administration, which include inhalants, enterals, topicals, ophtalmics, otics, and parenterals.

INHALANTS

Inhalants are inhaled through the patient's nose and/or mouth into the lungs. These medications are not required to be sterile (meaning administered without the presence of a pyrogen or particulates), since these substances may be naturally occurring in the patient. The respiratory system naturally filters the air before the air enters the lungs through the presence of nose hair.

ENTERALS

enteral
a method of nutrient delivery in which medication is given directly into the gastrointestinal tract

The second form of administration is the **enteral** route. The enteral route includes all of the gastrointestinal tract from the mouth to the intestines. The different forms of medication include tablets, capsules, solutions, elixirs, oral suspensions, lozenges, and suppositories. This route of administration also does not have to be sterile because of the body's natural defense system. Most enteral medications are taken orally, which means that unless they are directly absorbed in the mouth, such as sublingual tablets, or absorbed in the large intestine, such as suppositories, the medication passes though the stomach. The stomach produces hydrochloric acid (HCl), which has a pH of approximately 2, creating a hostile environment for most pyrogens. If any particulates are present, they are not absorbed in the small intestine and are passed through the body as a waste product.

TOPICALS

Topicals are usually placed on the skin and the medication is absorbed. Topicals include patches, ointments, creams, pastes, and liniments. The integumentary system, or skin, is another one of the body's defense systems; it acts as a covering to prevent pyrogens and particulates from entering the body. So again, most topicals do not have to be sterile. However, when the integumentary system is significantly compromised, such as in severe burn and surgical patients, topical preparations must be sterile. In these cases, the skin either cannot provide adequate protection or is physically not present to protect the body from the addition of pyrogens and/or particulates.

OPHTHALMICS AND OTICS

Ophthalmics and otics are drops or ointments that are specifically compounded for the eyes or ears. The otics are not considered sterile medications because they are administered externally. The ear, compared with the eye, has a better defense system to help combat pryogens and particulates.

Ophthalmics, however, must be sterile because all medications placed in the eye are readily absorbed—including pyrogens. Particulates can cause irritations or even be responsible for a scratched cornea.

PARENTERALS

The **parenteral** route is useful when the patient is unable to take medications by mouth, for whatever reason. It's also used in emergency treatments when rapid absorption is essential. Medications given by parenteral injection typically have a quicker onset of action. This route can be used to correct fluid and electrolyte imbalances and to provide nutrition when the patient cannot take food by mouth or feeding tube. The parental route can also be effective for local anesthetic effects in surgery. Infection becomes a risk due to the skin puncture; therefore, the use of aseptic technique is required. There are several different routes of parenteral injections. Of these, subcutaneous, intramuscular, and intravenous are the most commonly used.

parenteral
administration via injection

In *subcutaneous injections*, the solution or suspension is injected underneath the skin. This route usually has a slower onset. The maximum volume that can be injected subcutaneously is 2 mL. Patients, especially insulin-dependent diabetics, can easily be taught how to self-administer this type of injection.

The *intramuscular (IM) route* is quicker-acting than the subcutaneous route. The medication is injected deep into a large muscle mass, such as the buttocks, thighs, and upper arms. Up to 2.5 mL can be given in this form of injection. The biggest disadvantage to IM injections is the pain that is normally associated with them.

The *intravenous (IV) route* is the fastest option where parenteral administration is concerned because medication is introduced directly into the bloodstream. This is the preferred route for medicines that are irritating, because they are quickly diluted. The IV route is not as limited to volume as the other parenteral routes.

There are three ways that IV medications can be administered. An initial dose, often referred to as a **bolus**, can be injected into the vein and administered over a short period of time. This will normally be written IVP, for *intravenous push*. It is generally used for a small volume (less than 250 mL).

bolus
an initial dose

Another type of IV injection is called a *continuous infusion*. This involves a larger volume of solution (250 mL or more) spread over a longer administration time at a constant flow rate.

Intermittent infusions are delivered through the same set to avoid another needle stick. These are usually smaller volumes of 500 mL or less, to be given over a shorter time span than a continuous infusion. This type of infusion is known as a **piggyback**, or rider, and will be written IVPB. Antibiotic injections given using the IV route are commonly piggybacked. Since they are given with additional fluids running at the same time, the IV antibiotics are further diluted and are less irritating to the vein.

piggyback
(IVPB) delivery of a secondary IV solution from an outside source into an IV line containing fluid from an existing line

The parenteral route of administration is the most dangerous route of administration because it bypasses the body's defense systems. The parenteral route is essentially administered directly to the body, and in some cases directly into a specific organ. If proper aseptic technique is not practiced, not only is the medication administered but also possible pyrogens and/or particulates. The addition of pyrogens and/or particulates directly into the patient's body, which may already be compromised, can cause immense health complications such as **phlebitis**, **sepsis**, or death.

phlebitis
inflammation of a vein

sepsis
the presence of organisms in the blood

The following are routes of parenteral administration:

- **Intradermal**—abbreviated ID. The medication or fluid is injected directly into the skin's dermal layer. Intradermal administration can be used for skin tests such as tuberculosis and allergy tests. Intradermal administration should not exceed volumes greater than 0.1 mL and should be administered using a large-gauge needle.
- **Subcutaneous**—abbreviated SC or SQ. The medication or fluid is injected underneath the cutaneous layer of skin. Subcutaneous administration can be used for slowly absorbed medications such as insulin, anticoagulants (such as heparin or enoxaparin), and some hormones. Subcutaneous administration should not exceed volumes greater than 2.0 mL and should be administered using a large-gauge needle.
- **Intramuscular**—abbreviated IM. The medication or fluid is administered into the muscle. Intramuscular injections are used for some antibiotics, vitamins, hormones, vaccinations, suspensions, and oil-based products. Intramuscular injections are used when seeking more prolonged drug effects. Intramuscular administration dosages range between 2.0 mL and 5.0 mL depending on the injection site. A large-gauge needle should be used, but the needle length should also

be taken into account so that the needle is long enough to pass through the dermal layers into the muscles.

- **Intracardiac**—abbreviated IC. The medication is injected directly into the cardiac muscle or the heart. This form of administration is used in emergencies. The most common intracardiac medication is epinephrine, which comes in a prefilled syringe.
- **Epidural**—The medication or fluid is injected directly into the epidural space. Epidurals can be used to help control patients' pain either postoperatively or perinatally. The epidural or dura mater space is the outside layer of the spinal cord. Epidurals usually contain a narcotic mixed with a numbing agent such as bupivacaine or ropivacaine in a base solution such as normal saline. It is very important to compound epidurals with preservative-free materials; the presence of preservatives can cause permanent paralysis because of the body's inability to break down preservatives in the epidural space.
- **Intrathecal**—abbreviated IT. The medication or fluid is injected directly into the subarachnoid space surrounding the spinal cord. The spinal fluid in this space is "free circulating" between the brain and the rest of the spinal cord. The subarachnoid space is where a spinal tap is done to check for the presence of meningitis. This is also where spinal anesthesia is done. Intrathecal injections may provide chemotherapy for a patient with a brain tumor or brain **metathesis**. Again, all intrathecal medication must be preservative-free to prevent permanent paralysis or impaired cerebral function.

metathesis
a mere change in place of a morbid substance, without removal from the body

- **Intravenous**—abbreviated IV. The fluid medication is directly administered into the vein. This route achieves rapid effects and is the most common parenteral route used. The intravenous route is not restricted to a certain amount of fluid administered, but often is restricted by the patient's physical state. In other words, an adult can generally receive more intravenous fluid than a pediatric or neonatal patient. A dehydrated patient can receive more intravenous fluid than a patient who is in congestive heart failure.

Medication can be administered intravenously through two main routes—through a peripheral line or through a central line. Peripheral line accesses are located in the extremities such as the arms, hands, and feet (Figure 1-1). Central lines are accessed in the main trunk of the body, such as the subaortic and femoral veins. Peripheral lines are the most common route of intravenous administration because they are often the easiest to put in. Most medications are aseptically compounded to be peripherally administered. Central lines are used for various reasons. Sometimes when the patient is very ill or has weak peripheral veins, a central line is the only way he will be able to receive intravenous medication. In other cases, the medication may be too caustic (chemotherapy agents) or too concentrated for administration (total parenteral nutrition [TPN] bags) for administration in a peripheral

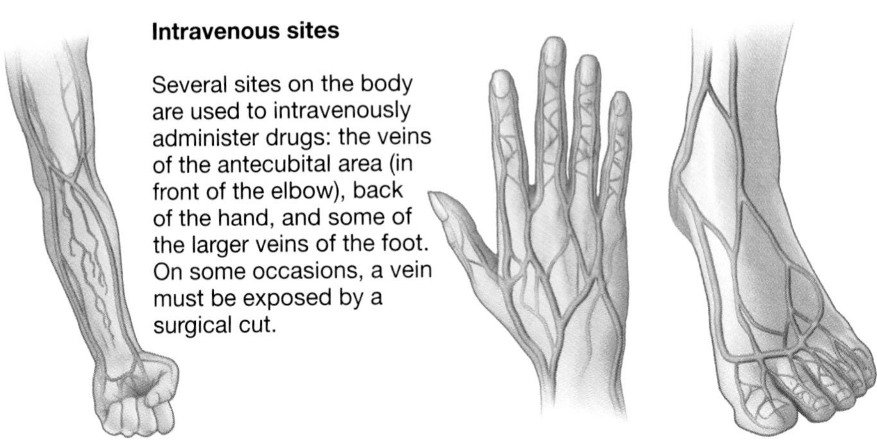

Figure 1-1 Intravenous administration sites

line. Peripheral veins are smaller in diameter compared to central veins. The central veins have more blood volume running through them compared to the peripheral veins, which allows more caustic and concentrated medications to be administered without damaging the blood vessels.

CONCLUSION

Sterile products are a vital component of modern pharmaceutical care; therefore, it is vital for pharmacy technicians to have a solid understanding and working knowledge of proper aseptic technique. Guidelines have been established for aseptic technique for the protection of both the patient and the personnel involved.

PROFILES OF PRACTICE

Depending on which state he is practicing in, a pharmacy technician may compound most, if not all, sterile products. The roles of pharmacists are becoming increasingly clinical-based: checking for possible allergies, duplicate orders, and correct dosages; serving as a reference for physicians and nurses; and many other clinical applications. With these increases in job responsibilities, the pharmacist needs help. More and more pharmacy technicians are receiving training and attending classes to learn about aseptic techniques and compounding practices.

States that require pharmacy technicians to be certified and/or require that technicians register with the state board of pharmacy usually give technicians more responsibility. In some progressive states, pharmacy technicians may compound any type of sterile product, including intravenous admixtures, ophthalmic medications, total parenteral nutrition (TPN) bags, and chemotherapy medications, all under the pharmacist's supervision, practicing what is universally known as aseptic technique.

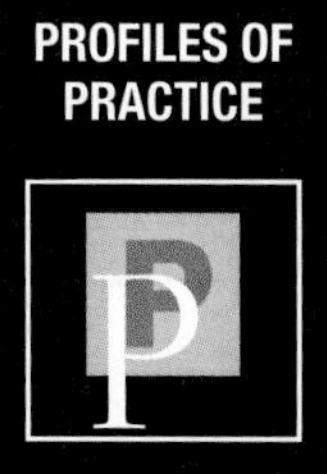

CHAPTER TERMS

bolus
an initial dose

enteral
a method of nutrient delivery in which medication is given directly into the gastrointestinal tract

metathesis
a mere change in place of a morbid substance, without removal from the body

parenteral
administration via injection

phlebitis
inflammation of a vein

piggyback
(IVPB) delivery of a secondary IV solution from an outside source into an IV line containing fluid from an existing line

pyrogen
a substance that produces fever

sepsis
the presence of organisms in the blood

CHAPTER REVIEW QUESTIONS

MATCHING

Please match the medication type with the correct route. Answers may be used more than once.

1. __________ inhalers
2. __________ ointments
3. __________ subcutaneous
4. __________ capsules
5. __________ irrigations
6. __________ tablets
7. __________ peripheral line
8. __________ intradermal
9. __________ central line
10. __________ eye drops

a. inhalants
b. enterals
c. topicals
d. ophthalmics and otics
e. parenterals
f. oral

MULTIPLE CHOICE

11. Why must medication given by the parenteral administration route be sterile or prepared aseptically? __________
    a. to prevent any possible contamination
    b. to prevent administration of contaminants to the patient
    c. intravenous administration bypasses all of the body's natural defense systems
    d. FDA regulations prevent aseptic compounding
    e. a, b, and c
    f. all of the above

MATCHING

Please choose the correct description for the parenteral route.

12. __________ intradermal
13. __________ subcutaneous
14. __________ intramuscular
15. __________ intracardiac
16. __________ epidural
17. __________ intrathecal
18. __________ intravenous

a. medication or fluid administered into the muscle
b. medication or fluid administered into the epidural space, which is the outer layer of the spinal cord
c. medication or fluid administered into a vein
d. medication administered into the cardiac muscle
e. medication or fluid administered into the subarachnoid space surrounding the spinal cord
f. medication or fluid administered under the dermis
g. medication or fluid administered into the dermis

Please indicate which of the following medications must be preservative-free.

19. __________ intradermal
20. __________ subcutaneous
21. __________ intramuscular
22. __________ intracardiac
23. __________ epidural
24. __________ intrathecal
25. __________ intravenous

a. may contain preservatives
b. may not contain preservatives

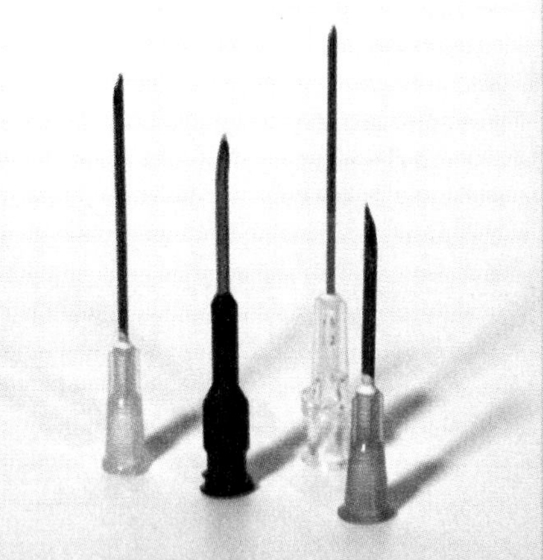

CHAPTER 2

Facilities, Garb, and Equipment

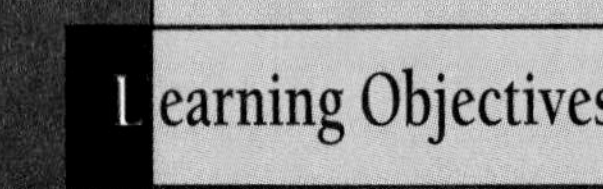

Learning Objectives

After completing this chapter, you should be able to:

- Explain how laminar flow biological safety cabinets contribute to infection control.
- Describe the difference among class 100, 1000, and 10,000 clean rooms.
- Explain the importance of aseptic technique in compounding.
- Explain the reason for each step in the proper procedure for cleaning a laminar flow biological safety cabinet.
- Describe the proper protective dress required in a clean room.

INTRODUCTION

In general, sterile products include products used for parenterals, ophthalmics, and select irrigations. The final product must be free from chemical and physical contaminants, accurately and correctly compounded, pharmaceutically elegant, pyrogen-free, and stable for its intended shelf-life. It must also be packaged in a manner that will ensure maintenance of its quality until used.

The area in which the compounding will take place is commonly referred to as a clean room. The equipment could differ from facility to facility. There are, however, universal standards regarding facilities, equipment, and dress. The mandatory requirements and related suggestions appear in good professional guidelines, such as those provided by the American Society of Health-System Pharmacists (ASHP). Each facility should have a more specific policy pertaining to its needs in addition to these universal guidelines.

Whatever practice setting the pharmacy technician spends his career in, it will require some form of clothing specific to the company. For preparing sterile products, however, the items that the pharmacy technician will be required to wear may include various types of coverings for the face, eyes, hands, feet, and other body parts.

Four key factors contribute to the preparation of high-quality sterile products: facilities, environmental control, components, and operators.

Facilities and Clean Room

The ASHP "Technical Assistance Bulletin on Quality Assurance for Pharmacy-Prepared Sterile Products" (1993) and United States Pharmacopeia (USP) Chapter 1206, "Sterile Drug Products for Home Use" (1995), provided directions for setting quality standards and practices for achieving them. Later, we will discuss USP 797 regulations (published in January 2004) and their impact on aseptic facilities, environmental control, components, and operators.

Facilities that perform aseptic compounding must have a designated area for this task. This area should be placed in a section of the facility where traffic is very limited and airflow is unrestricted. Only designated personnel should enter this space, and only for the purpose of aseptic preparations. The room should be large enough to accommodate necessary equipment, such as the laminar airflow hood (LAH), and to provide for the proper storage of drugs and supplies under appropriate conditions of temperature, light, moisture, sanitation, ventilation, and security. The LAH should be inside the aseptic preparation area, while storage shelves, sinks, refrigerators, and so on should be kept in a separate but close area. This designated area should contain all the criteria for being a clean room.

Clean rooms are rooms in which the air quality, temperature, and humidity are highly regulated in order to greatly reduce the risk of cross-contamination. The air in a clean room is repeatedly filtered to remove dust particles, **particulates**, and other impurities.

particulates
small matter

Most institutional IV rooms are clean rooms. The measure of the air quality of a clean room is described in Federal Standard 209D. Clean rooms are rated as follows:

- Class 10,000: no more than 10,000 particles larger than 0.5 micron in any given cubic foot of air
- Class 1000: no more than 1000 particles larger than 0.5 micron in any given cubic foot of air
- Class 100: no more than 100 particles larger than 0.5 micron in any given cubic foot of air

The clean room usually has only one door, which should remain closed when not in use. It is a positive-pressure room, which means that when the door is opened, air will flow out of the clean room. It is designed to keep particulates from flowing into the room when the door is in use. There should be no cardboard items in the clean room either, to help limit free-floating particles. (See Figure 2-1).

The purpose of the positive pressure is to keep unfiltered or dirty air from entering the clean room where the clean air is. The air in a clean room is purified so that it is cleaner than the air in the rest of the pharmacy and/or

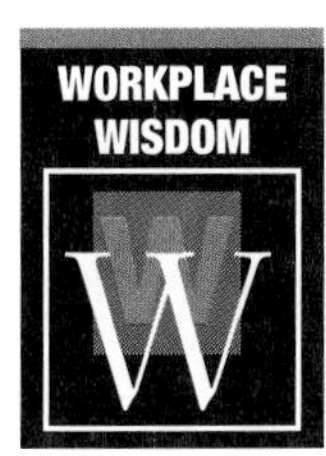

The environmental control of air is of concern because room air may be highly contaminated. For example, sneezing produces 100,000–200,000 aerosol droplets that can then attach to dust particles. These contaminated particles may be present in the air for weeks.

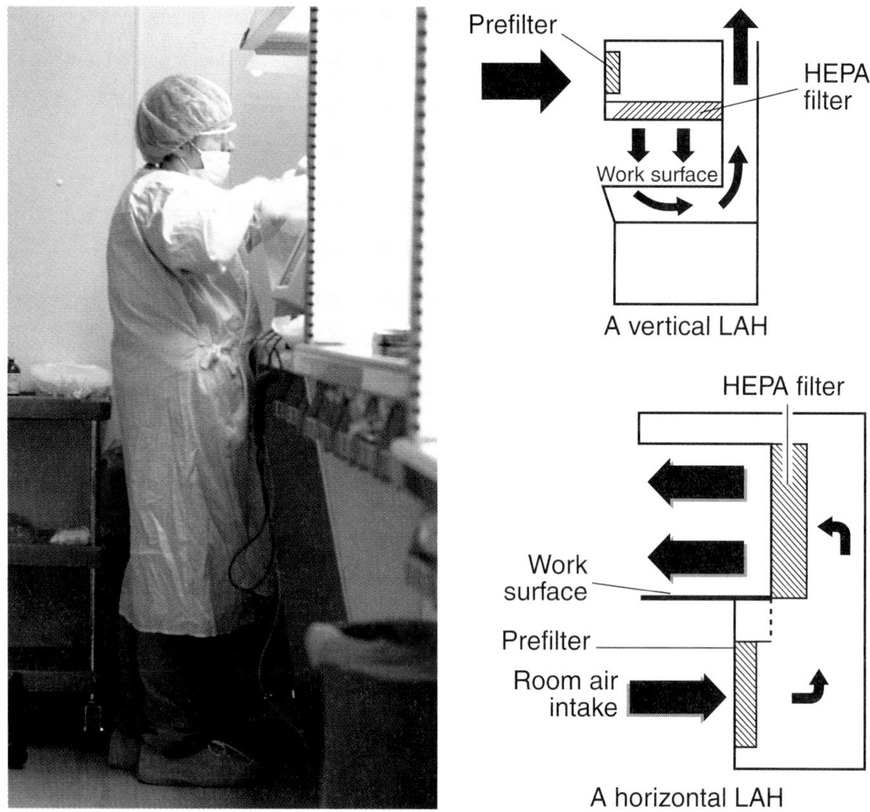

Figure 2-1 Clean room

Figure 2-2 Positive pressure airflow

hospital. The cleaner the air, the less chance that contaminants will be introduced into a sterile product (Figure 2-2).

Supplies necessary for aseptic preparation, such as syringes, needles, and alcohol swabs, should be kept to a minimum. These supplies are usually close by in a cart of some sort or in storage near the hood. In a clean room, furniture such as counters is made of stainless steel, which is easy to clean with 70% isopropyl alcohol and is particulate-free. In addition to all the equipment and other surfaces in this area, the floors should be cleaned and sanitized daily, working from the cleanest area outward.

USP 797

In January 2004, USP issued a set of new and stringent regulations regarding aseptic preparations. Included in this set of documents is a new approach to facility design, microbial contamination risk levels, personnel training and evaluation, clean room atmosphere, proper dress, quality assurance, validation, and monitoring.

For many years, facilities have operated under guidelines such as the ones set by the USP and ASHP as previously mentioned. USP 797 expands on many of those previous criteria. Although USP 797 has been officially released, it is constantly being reevaluated and may be subject to revisions as other factors are considered.

For facilities, USP 797 states that the surfaces of all ceilings, walls, floors, shelving, cabinets, and work surfaces in the buffer room and/or **anteroom** should be smooth, free from cracks and crevices, and nonshedding, making them easy to clean and sanitize (Figure 2-3). The anteroom is a separate area close to the preparation area where gowning and hand washing take place. Junctures of ceilings to walls, walls to walls, and floors to walls should be covered or caulked to make them easier to clean. The areas should have no dust-collecting ledges, pipes, or similar surfaces. Work surfaces should be durable and smooth and made of stainless steel or molded plastic. Carts should be of stainless steel wire or sheet construction with good-quality, cleanable casters and should be restricted to the controlled area.

anteroom
the room located right outside the clean room; it is a low-particulate room, which means that it should not contain paper, boxes, or high-particulate matter. Food and drink should not be allowed in this room

THE AIRFLOW HOOD

In the 1960s, due to the increased need for clean air in the industry, airflow hoods (also known as *clean benches* or *laminar flow cabinets*) were first developed to provide product protection for small-scale experimental procedures. Today, airflow hoods are used at a number of facilities and labs for all types of sterile procedures. Pharmacy technicians work with airflow hoods while mixing IV or chemotherapy solutions.

An airflow hood provides a controlled environment in which levels of particulates, microbes, and contaminants of all kinds are regulated and kept to a minimum by constant air filtration. The hood creates a particle-free working environment by taking in air through a filtration system and exhausting it across a work surface in a laminar or unidirectional airstream.

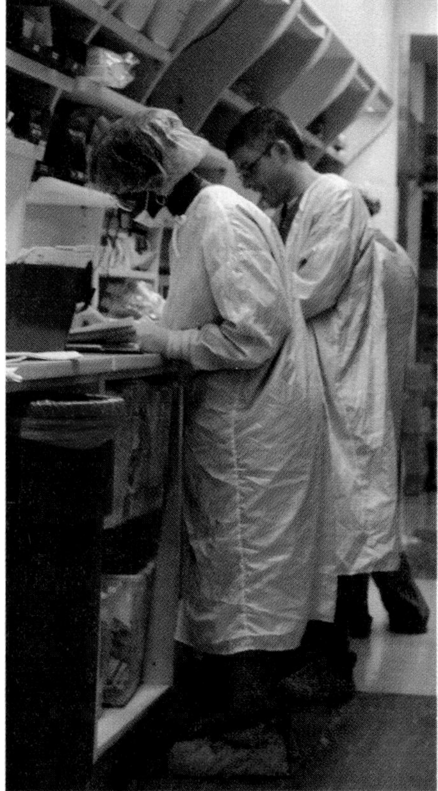

Figure 2-3 Anteroom

Commonly, the filtration system consists of a prefilter and a high-efficiency particulate air (HEPA) filter. Because the air within the cabinet does not contain any airborne particles (Figure 2-3), it is also sterile. The airflow hood is usually enclosed on the sides and kept under constant positive pressure in order to prevent infiltration of contaminated room air.

There are two main types of airflow hoods—the laminar airflow hood (LAH) and the vertical airflow hood, or biological safety cabinet (BSC). The airflow in the LAH flows horizontally from the back of the hood toward the front of the hood, whereas the airflow in the BSC flows vertically downward from the top of the hood toward the work surface. Each hood is designed to sterilize through filtration using a HEPA filter.

The function of airflow hoods is twofold:

- to filter bacteria and other particulate matter from the air, and
- to maintain a constant airflow out of the hood to prevent entry of contaminants.

Laminar Airflow Hood

All aseptic compounding should take place in the LAH (Figure 2-4). The LAH has a prefilter in the front of the hood that removes any large contaminants from the room air. The prefilter should be changed monthly and documented. After the air has been filtered once through the prefilter, it travels to the back of the hood where it is filtered again in the HEPA filter. The HEPA filter removes particles that are 2 microns and larger. That is almost all bacteria, fungi, and viruses. The filtered air is then blown horizontally toward the front of the hood. The HEPA filter is not changed but should be tested every six months for efficiency. The LAH must be turned on for at least 30 min before any aseptic compounding can take place.

Biological Safety Cabinet

Hazardous compounding (chemotherapy) takes place in the BSC (Figure 2-5). There are two main types of BSC, which differ based on where the filtered air from the BSC is exhausted. Both hoods have four sides with an 8- to 12-in. opening in the front. A sliding glass front can be brought down to the proper opening level.

The opening in the front allows the room air to be sucked into the BSC grills, which are located in the front and back of the inside of the hood's work surface area. This air is then filtered and circulated to the HEPA filter, which then filters the air to 0.3 micron. The filtered air is blown from the top of the hood vertically downward to the work surface area. The air is then filtered again and either eliminated back into the room air or to an outside vent. As with the LAH, the HEPA filter should be tested every six months.

Cleaning the Hood

germicidal
describes an agent that kills pathogenic microorganisms

Bacteria and surface contamination can be expected, even if it is not visible. Written standard procedures should be developed and followed for cleaning and sanitizing all surfaces within the controlled area. As mentioned previously, water and 70% isopropyl alcohol or other **germicidal** products are typ-

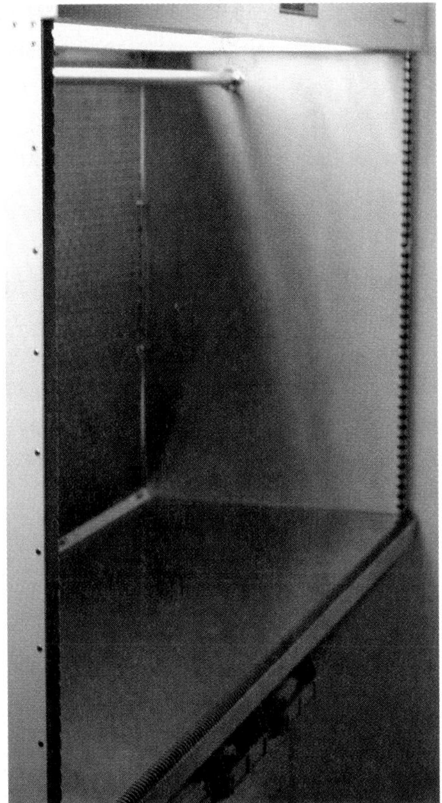

Figure 2-4 Laminar airflow hood

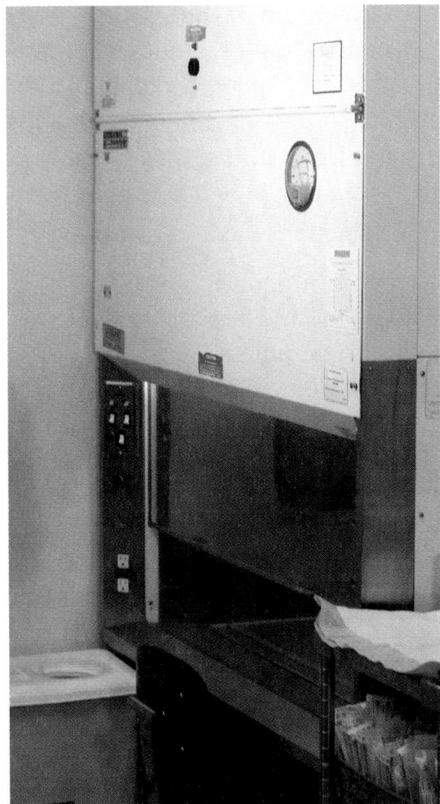

Figure 2-5 Biological safety cabinet

ically used. All reusable cleaning tools, such as mops, should be restricted to the controlled area and thoroughly cleaned and sanitized after each use.

A thorough cleaning of the hood must be done at least a minimum of every 8 hr or when the hood becomes dirty. The hood can never be cleaned too much. Anyone who compounds should wipe down the surface area frequently. A compounder should wipe down the surface area when finished preparing one type of product and before compounding another. For example, when finished preparing a penicillin-based product, the compounder should wipe down the hood before mixing another product. This is because some patients may be allergic to penicillin, and in aseptic compounding one goal is to prevent cross-contaminants from entering a product.

The procedure for properly cleaning the hood is as follows (See Figure 2-6):

1. Wash the entire hood walls and surface with sterile water to remove salt, starch, sugar, and/or proteins.
2. Soak stubborn spots for 5-10 min, then wipe clean.
3. To disinfect, wipe all the surfaces of the hood with 70% isopropyl alcohol using lint-free fabric. Alcohol disinfects the hood in the drying process known as **desiccation**. If the alcohol is not dry, then the surface is not clean. The idea behind the lint-free fabric is to reduce the amount of lint particles or other contaminants that can be brought into the

desiccation
the act of dehydrating or removing water content

clean room. If the specially designed paper towels are not available, you may use gauze. Under no circumstances should you use regular or industrial paper towels; they produce excessive lint.

4. Wipe top to bottom on the sides and back wall and left to right on the flat work surface area. Wipe down all parts inside the hood, such as the pole and the brackets holding the pole.
5. Document the hood cleaning at least once per shift or every 8 hr.

Aseptic compounding is best performed with high-quality components and equipment and knowledgeable personnel. Maintaining an aseptic environment is equipment-, labor-, and management-intensive, but it is not technically challenging. The goal of the aseptic environment is to prevent cross-contamination. Since contaminating bacteria are found everywhere, including fingertips, bench tops, and countertops, it is important to minimize contact with these contaminating surfaces.

It is highly important for the pharmacy technician to be aware of and practice proper cleaning procedures as well as aseptic techniques. Cleaning equipment after each use is standard practice regardless of where the compounding is being done.

OTHER SUPPLIES

Other supplies commonly found in or near a clean room for use include the following:

- Sink with hot and cold running water convenient to the compounding area
- Appropriate disposal or sharps containers for used needles, syringes, and so on, and, if applicable, for infectious wastes and cytotoxic waste from the preparation of chemotherapy agents
- refrigerator/freezer with a thermometer
- infusion devices, if appropriate
- disposable needles, syringes, and other supplies needed for aseptic admixture
- disinfectant cleaning solutions
- hand-washing agent with germicidal action
- disposable, lint-free towels or wipes
- appropriate filters and filtration equipment
- disposable masks, caps, gowns, and sterile disposable gloves if applicable

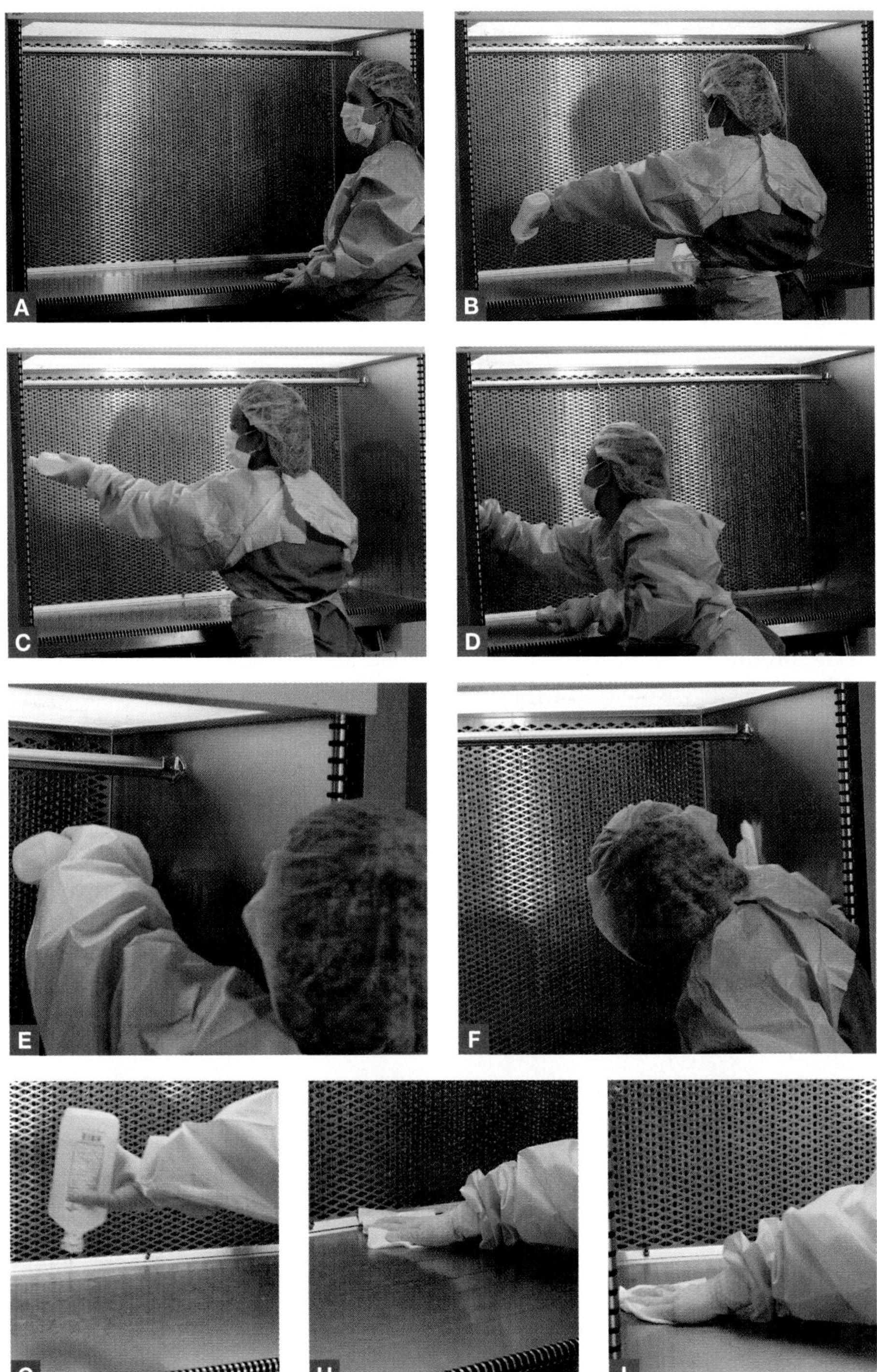

Figure 2-6 Cleaning the LAH

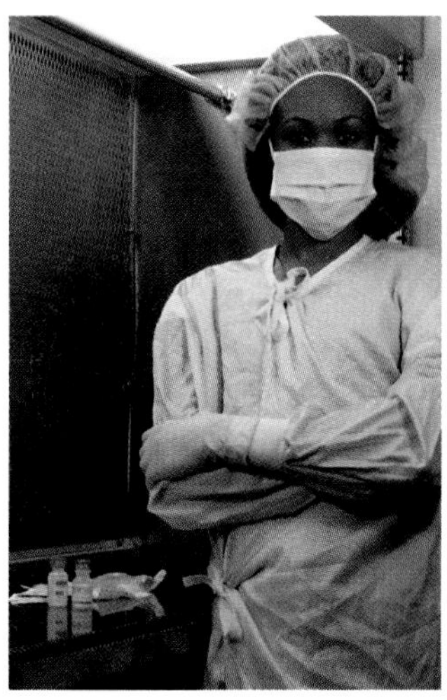

Figure 2-7 IV technician

The Dressings (Garb)

Clean garments that are relatively particulate-free should be worn when working in the sterile preparation area.

PERSONAL ATTIRE WITHIN THE IV AREA

Personnel who enter the sterile product preparations area should wear clean hospital scrub uniforms or surgical gowns. This applies to everyone entering the sterile products area, whether working under the hood or checking IVs. Disposable surgical gowns can be worn when working under the hood. The gowns should be removed before leaving the IV room and should be disposed of at the end of each shift or upon contamination. Everyone in this environment must wear a disposable hair cover. Surgical masks are required for anyone with a cough, a cold, or any other type of transmittable illness. Men with facial hair must wear masks while working under the hood (Figure 2-7).

GOWNING

The following is a list of dressing supplies that may be required to prepare sterile products. Not all supplies are needed at all times. You should check with your facility to determine proper dress for different situations.

Supplies

- **Hair cover** a surgical cap to cover the hair; prevents addition of extra particulates in the clean room (Figure 2-8).
- **Shoe covers** cover the shoes; prevent addition of extra particulates and prevent any dirt from falling off of the shoes in the clean room (Figure 2-9).

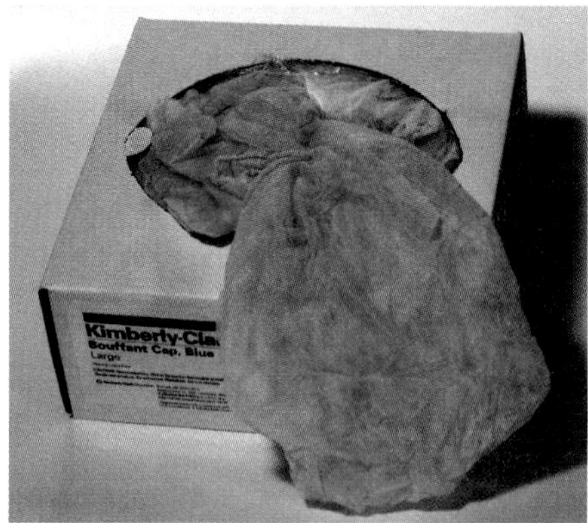

Figure 2-8 Hair cover

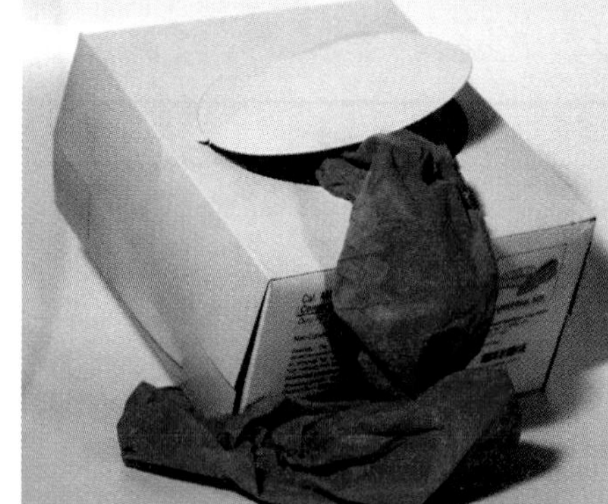

Figure 2-9 Shoe covers

- **Gloves** cover the hands; prevent the transfer of contaminants from places such as under the fingernails. Gloves also protect any wounds on the hands such as minor scratches (Figure 2-10).
- **Mask** covers any facial hair; prevents addition of extra particulates (Figure 2-11).

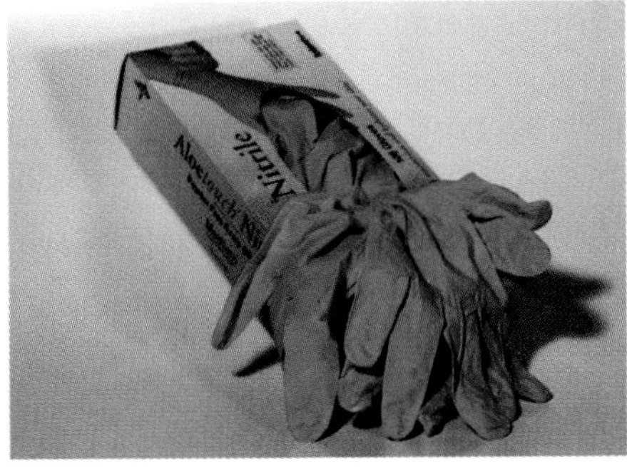

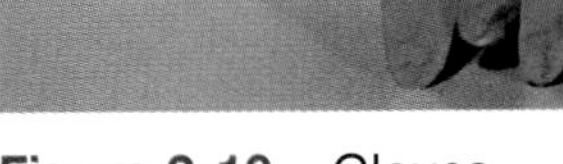

Figure 2-10 Gloves

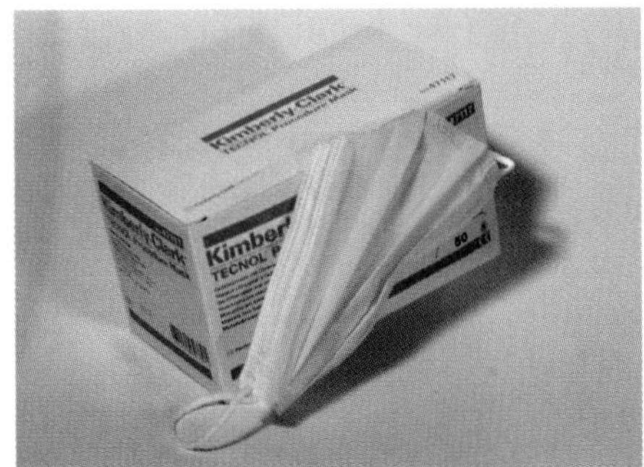

Figure 2-11 Masks

- **Gown** covers street clothes before entering the clean room; prevents addition of extra particulates (Figure 2-12).
- **Scrubs** Scrubs are designed to be low particulate and can be sterilized by the institution. Scrubs are the preferred clothing in a clean room. However, in a clean 100 room, only scrubs may be worn (Figure 2-13).

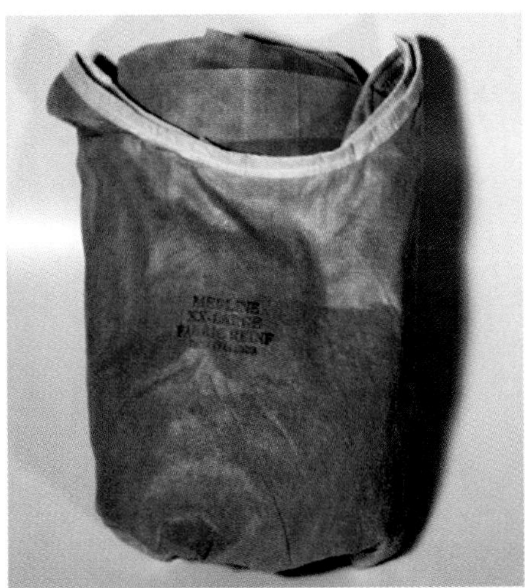

Figure 2-12 Gown

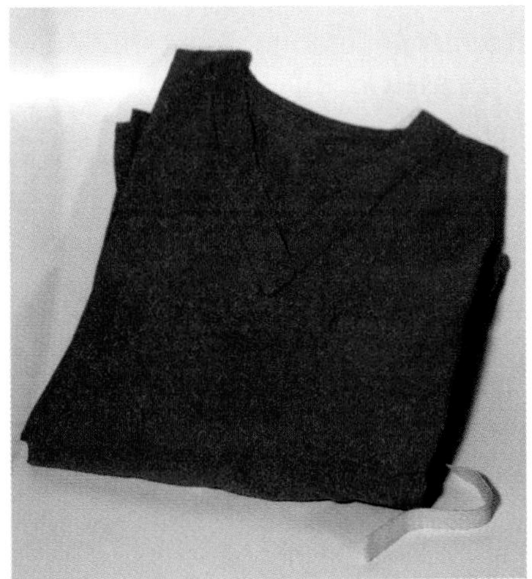

Figure 2-13 Scrubs

Gowning Procedure

Before working under the hood, the employee should be properly gowned.

- Before entering the clean room, first put on disposable hair and shoe covers. All hair must be completely covered, including facial hair such as beards, mustaches, and goatees. Specially designed garments are made specifically for these areas that need to be covered.
- Put on a disposable surgical gown, which usually closes and ties in back. Gowns, hair covers, and shoe covers should not be worn outside the clean room. If any of these are worn outside the pharmacy, the garment is considered contaminated and must be disposed of, requiring new gowning material. However, gowns may be reworn

during a shift if they have not been contaminated. Still, gowns are disposed of at the end of each shift.

- Gloves must extend over the cuff of the gown and be washed according to the hand-washing procedures.

For working with sterile preparations that are noncytotoxic, this is all you need. With hazardous materials such as chemotherapy preparations, the dressings are slightly different but similar in nature. This will be discussed in Chapter 8.

Compounding Supplies

There are numerous supplies needed for compounding and a discussion of each follows.

ALCOHOL PADS

Alcohol pads are kept close by at all times during preparation and used constantly for wiping down such things as vial tops (Figure 2-14).

NEEDLES

Needles are used to puncture containers and withdraw or inject fluid. There is a variety of different needle gauges and lengths (Figure 2-15).

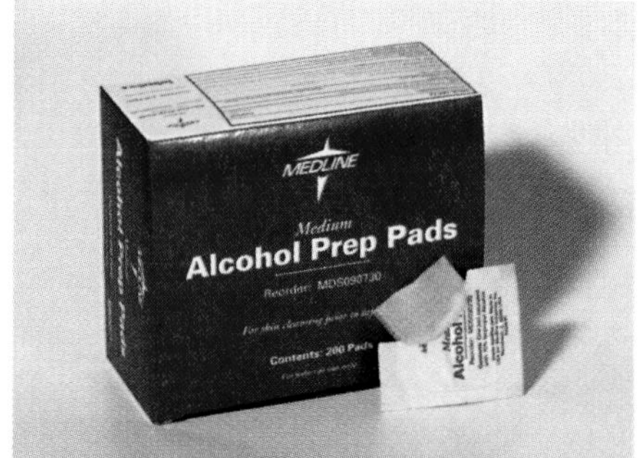

Figure 2-14 Alcohol pads

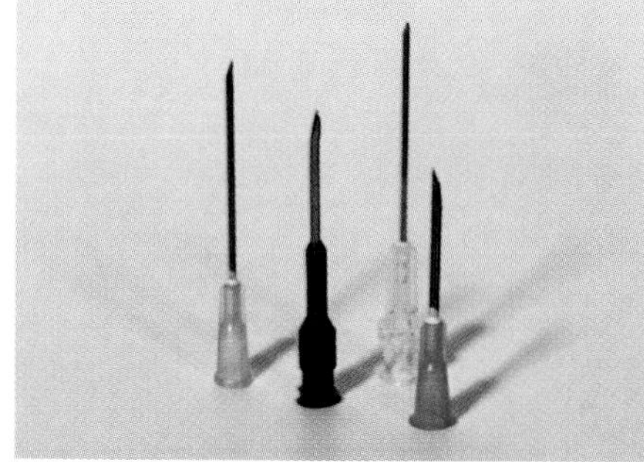

Figure 2-15 Needles (various)

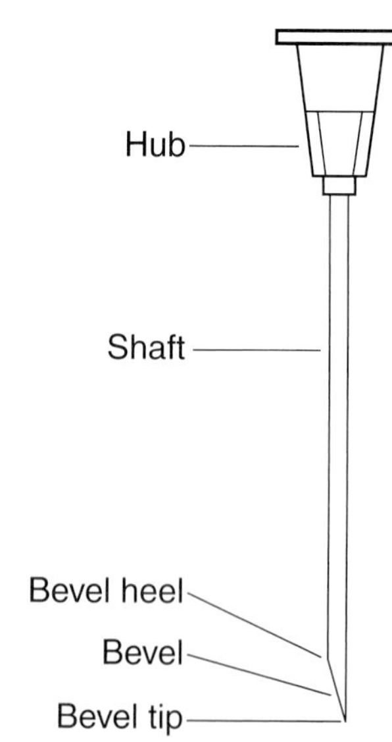

Figure 2-16 Parts of a needle

Parts of a Needle (Figure 2-16)

- **Lumen** the hollow space inside a needle
- **Bevel** the sharp pointed end of the needle
- **Heel** the opposite of the bevel; the rounded bottom part of the needle
- **Hub** the part of the needle that attaches to the syringe

Parts of a Syringe (Figure 2-17)

- **Tip** where the needle is attached to the syringe. This part should never be touched by anything.
- **Barrel** the part of the syringe where it is usually held. The barrel is where the fluid is held (on the inside). The barrel has the measurement gradations on it.

- **Plunger** slides in and out of the barrel. The plunger should never be touched except on the very end. If the plunger is touched and the plunger goes back into the barrel, the inside of the barrel is now contaminated.

Two Types of Needles

- **Luer-lock** the needle has to be physically screwed onto the syringe (Figure 2-18).
- **Slip tip** the needle slides onto the end of the syringe (Figure 2-19).

Needle Length

Different types of injections need different lengths of needles. Sizes may range from $\frac{3}{8}$ in. to $3\frac{1}{2}$ in. or longer (Figure 2-20).

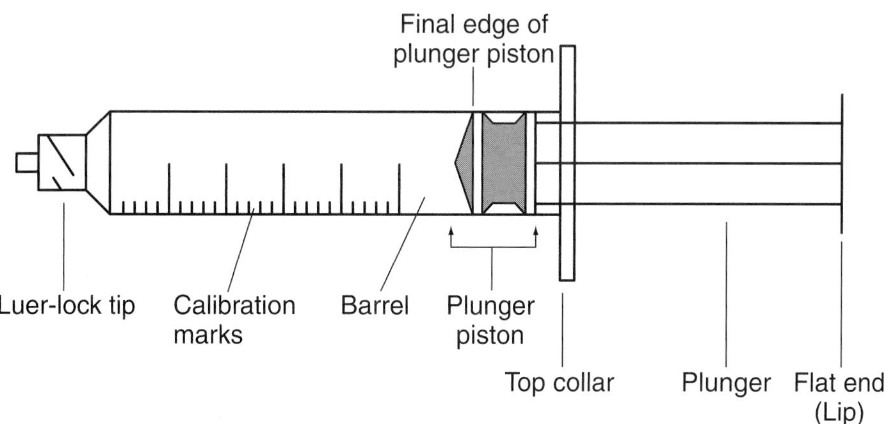

Figure 2-17 Parts of a syringe

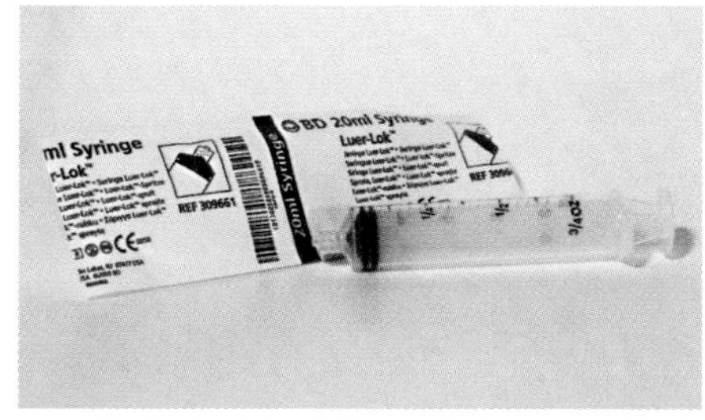

Figure 2-18 Luer-lock syringe

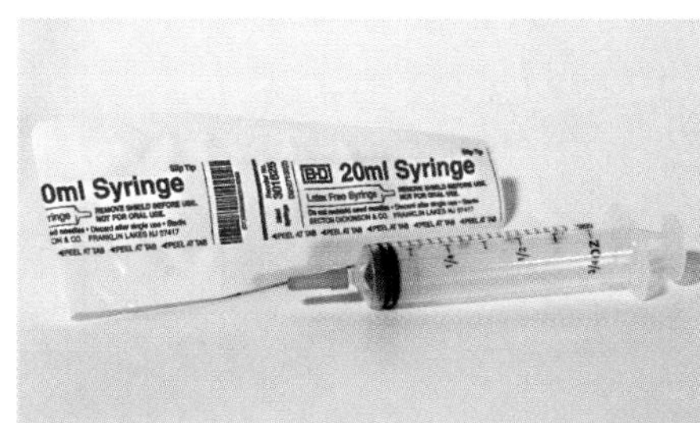

Figure 2-19 Slip tip

Gauge

Gauge refers to the size of the opening of a needle. The larger the gauge of a needle, the smaller the opening. Example, a 25-gauge needle has a very small opening, whereas an 18-gauge needle has a large opening. Needle gauges may range from 28 to 16 (Figure 2-21).

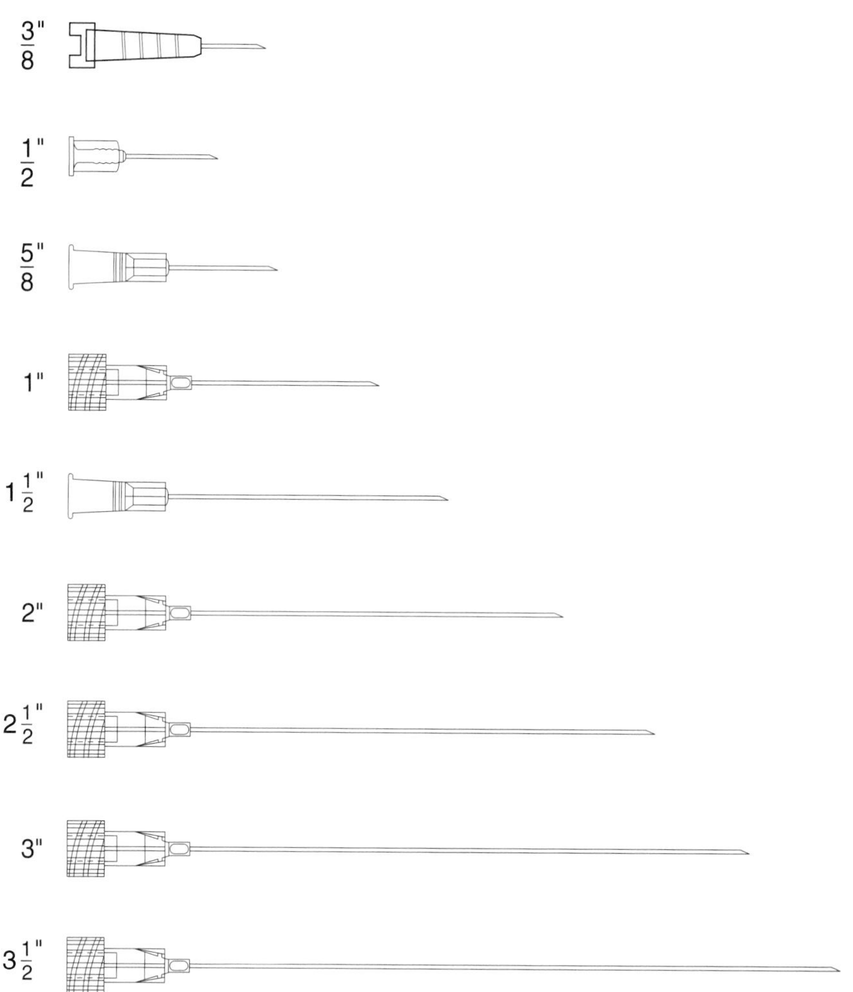

Figure 2-20 Needle lengths

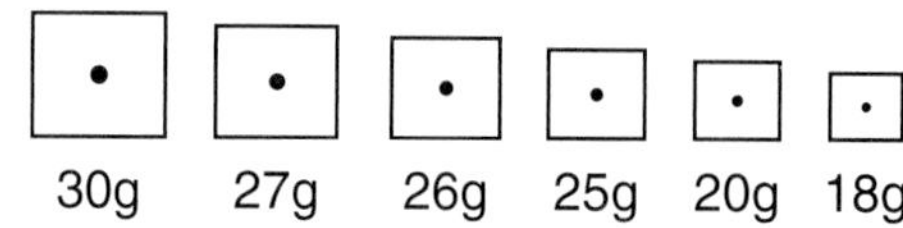

Figure 2-21 Needle gauges

MISCELLANEOUS

- **Ampule** a sealed container, usually made of glass, containing a sterile medicinal solution, or a powder to be made up in solution, to be used for injection.
- **Single dose vial (SDV)** a vial that contains no preservatives once the container is entered, contaminants may have been introduced and the container is no longer sterile.
- **Sticky mats** mats placed on the floor in the entrance from the anteroom to the clean room. The mats have multiple layers of sticky sheets that can be removed one layer at a time. The mats remove any particulates that may be carried into the clean room on the bottoms of the feet.
- **Vials** Vials that have preservatives will stay sterile for an extended period of time. The vial's expiration date is determined by the manufacturer's testing. Please read the package insert on the vial before giving it an expiration date (Figure 2-22).
- **Filters** Filters are used to remove air, bacteria, fungi, and particulates from a solution. There are three main types:
  - **Membrane filters** used to remove particulates from a solution. They are attached to the syringe and used as a form of sterilization (Figure 2-23).
  - **Depth filters** (filter needles and straws)—used to remove glass shards from a solution. The filter is part of the needle and can be used only once (Figure 2-24).
  - **In-line filters** used as part of the patient's IV set to filter solutions before they enter the patient (Figure 2-25).

vial
a small bottle or container that holds products such as injectable medications

Figure 2-22 Vials (various)

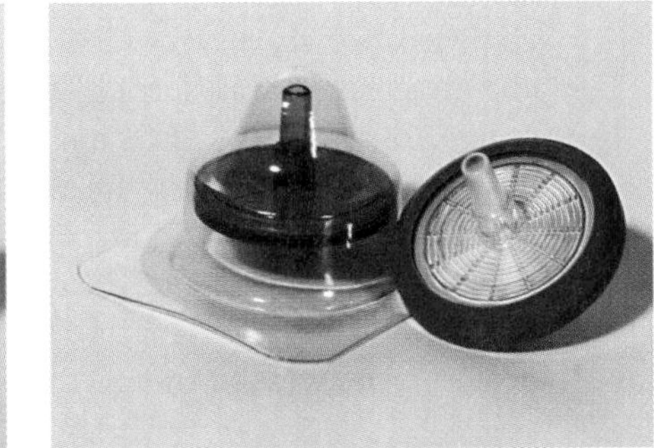

Figure 2-23 Membrane filter

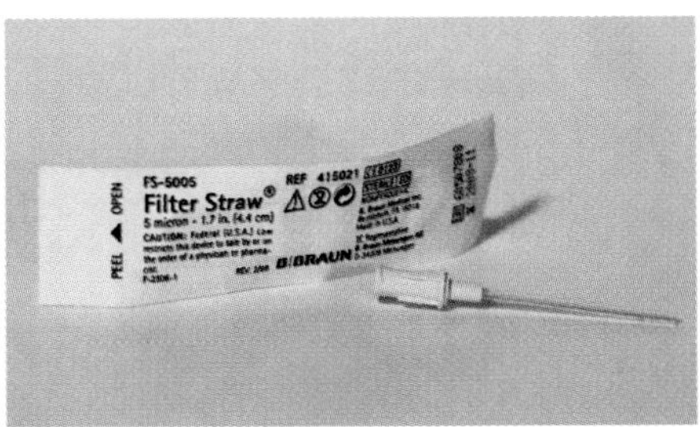

Figure 2-24 Filter straw

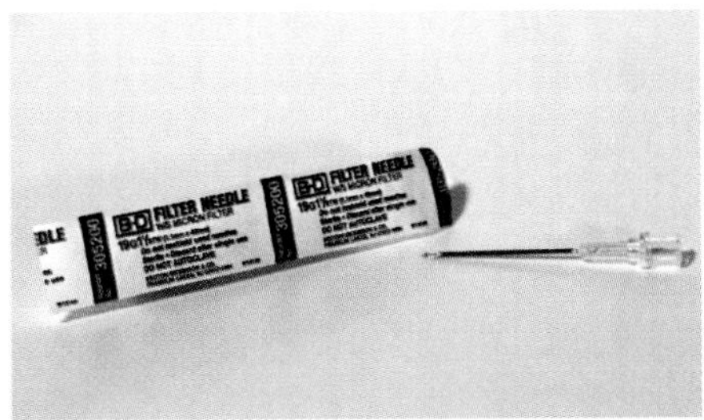

Figure 2-25 Filter needle

- **IV tubing** IV tubing is used to transfer fluid either from an IV bag to another container or from an IV bag to a patient (Figure 2-26).
- **Primary tubing** Primary tubing is used to transfer IV fluid from an IV bag or bottle to a patient. It is usually used by the nursing staff in most facilities; however, if the pharmacy's responsibility is to "prime the tubing," it will use primary tubing. Primary tubing also has many ports so that more than one IV can be administered at the same time (Figure 2-27).

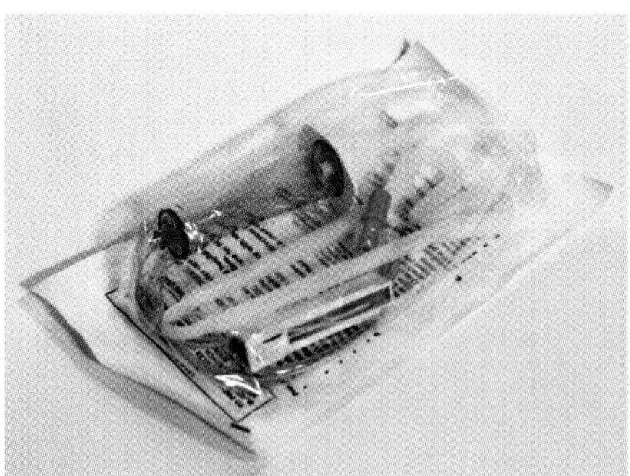

Figure 2-26 IV tubing

Figure 2-27 Non-vented tubing

- **Vented tubing** Vented tubing is used primarily by pharmacies to transfer the contents of one container to another container for administration. This tubing can transfer only one solution at a time (Figure 2-28).
- **Empty evacuated containers (EECs)** EECs are glass containers that are vacuumed or have a great negative pressure (Figure 2-29). They come in a variety of sizes (150 mL, 250 mL, 500 mL, and 1000 mL) and are great for transferring large volumes from one container to another. Advantages of EECs include the following: There are several different types of glass; they are stronger than plastic; they can be autoclaved, it is easier to inspect the contents, and some are amber-colored for light-sensitive medications. Some disadvantages are that they can be very heavy and hard to handle; have to be vented; and have rubber stoppers, which can lead to coring.

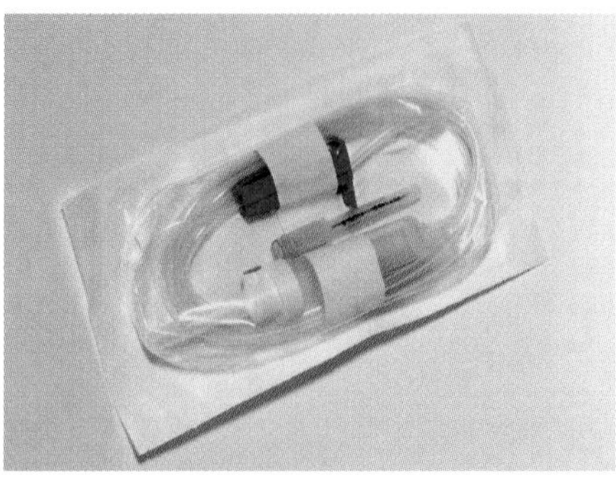

Figure 2-28 Vented tubing

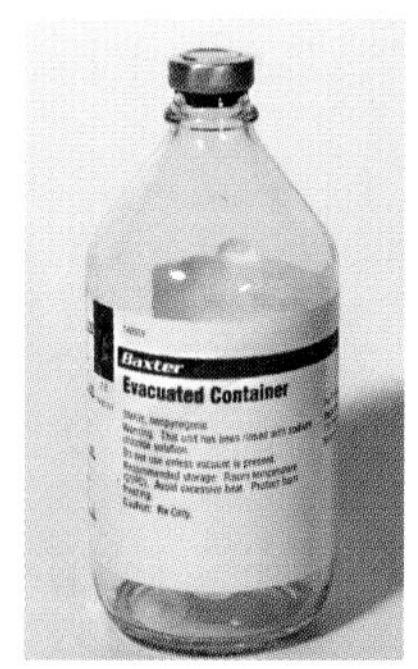

Figure 2-29 EEC

- **Viaflex bags** are empty plastic IV bags (Figure 2-30). Viaflex bags bags have several advantages compared to glass bottles: They are lighter and easier to handle, are less likely to break, and do not require an exchange of air. Some disadvantages are permeability to gases and vapor, leaching of the constituents of the container to the internal contents, transmission of light, masking of chemical incompatibilities, and inability to be thermally sterilized, as they would melt.

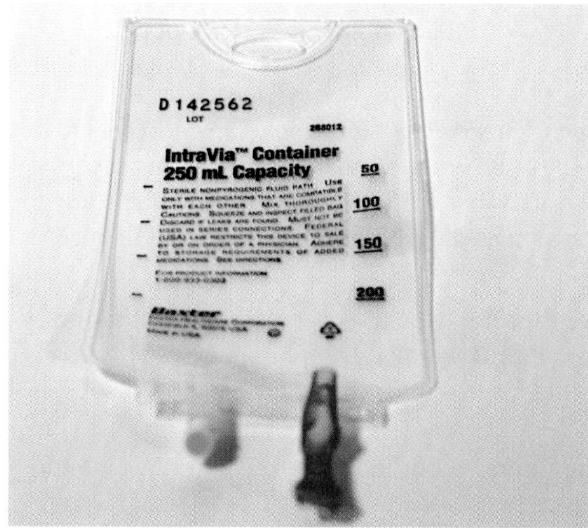

Figure 2-30 Viaflex bag

- **Leur-to-leur connectors** This is a needleless system that is very useful when transferring the contents of one syringe to another (Figure 2-31).
- **Dispensing pins** Dispensing pins are a needleless system that allows the contents of a vial to be removed using a leur-lock syringe. The dispensing pins are also vented, which allows easy transfer of material (Figure 2-32).
- **Intravenous piggybacks (IVPB)** IVPB consists of sterile IV fluid, usually NS or D5W, in a small IV bag to which additives are added. These IV bags are usually given on a schedule as opposed to a continuous drip.
- **Large volumes (LV)** LV bags are usually hydration, replacement, or nutrition bags. These IV bags are run continuously.

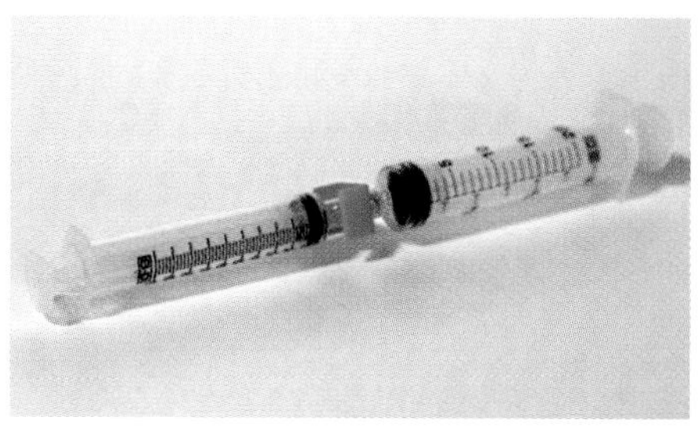

Figure 2-31 Leur-to-leur connector

Figure 2-32 Dispensing pin

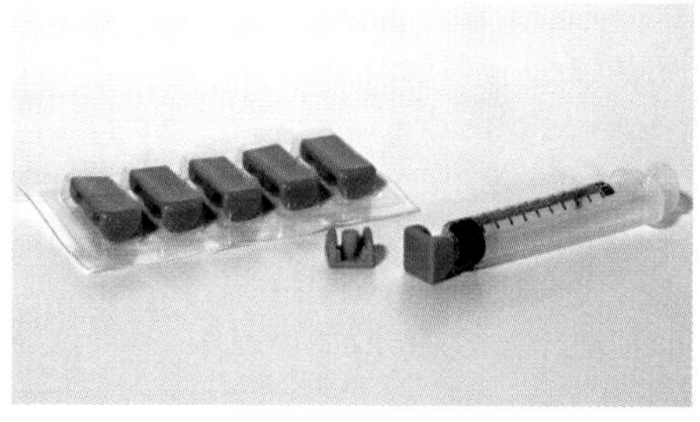

Figure 2-33 Syringe cap

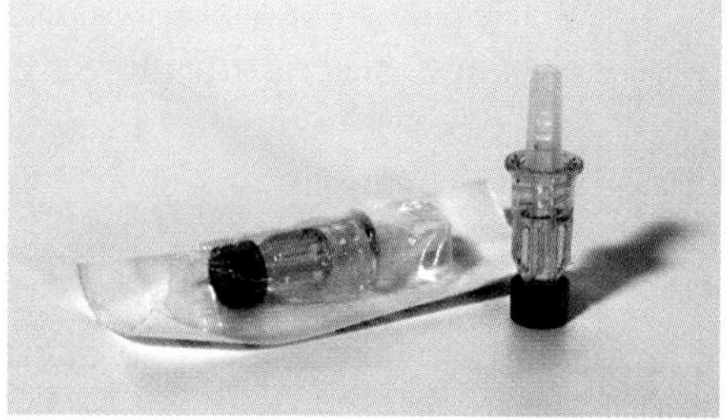

Figure 2-34 Port adapter

- **Mini-bags or Advantage** This IVPB system allows an entire vial to be aseptically attached to the IVPB without mixing the contents of the vial. These IVPBs can be activated or mixed when the nurse is ready to administer them. The advantage is that they allow for a much longer expiration date.
- **Syringe caps** Syringe caps are used to cover the ends of syringes until they are ready for administration. The pharmacy usually removes the needles so there is less of a chance for needle sticks (Figure 2-33).
- **Port adapters (male adapters)** Port adapters are external IV additive ports that can be attached to the IV additive post of an IV bag. These are great when several different additives are to be added to the IV bag. This way all of the needle sticks occur in the port adapter, while the IV additive port only has one needle stick (Figure 2-34).
- **IVA seals (foil port covers)** IVA seals are used to cover the additive port of an IV bag after the additives have been added. The IVA seal creates a physical barrier to prevent contamination of the IV bag (Figure 2-35).
- **Auxiliary labels** Auxiliary labels help keep the aseptically compounded medication in the correct storage requirements. Examples of auxiliary labels are "protect from light," "refrigerate," and "do not refrigerate."
- **Dark bags** These amber bags are placed over an IV, syringe, or bottle to keep the medication out of direct light.

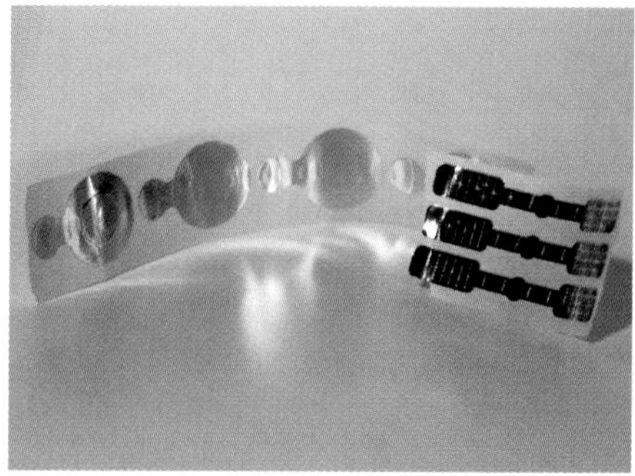

Figure 2-35 IVA seal

- **Red sharps containers** Red sharps containers are where any blood products, syringes, needles, glass, or broken glass waste products are thrown away. Red sharps containers require special disposal (Figure 2-36).
- **Vented spike adapters** Vented spike adapters are used to vent glass bottles that are attached to tubing (Figure 2-37).

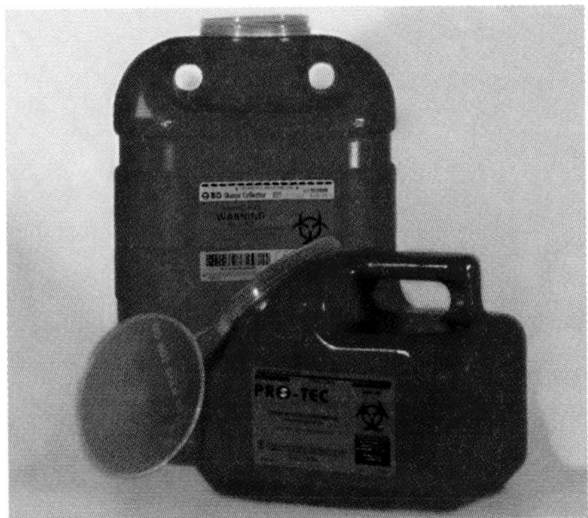

Figure 2-36 Sharps container

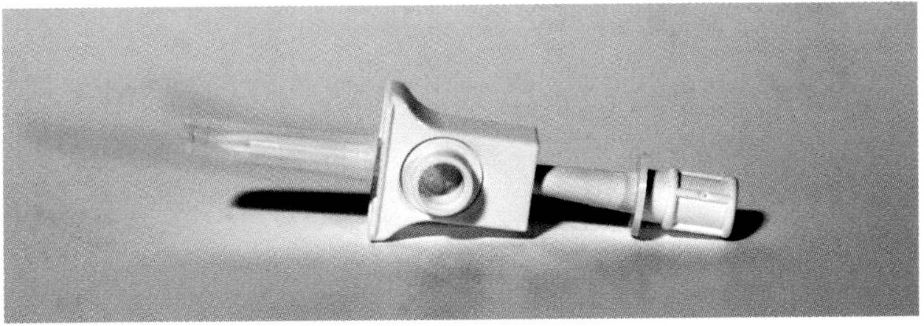

Figure 2-37 Vented spike adapter

OTHER EQUIPMENT

Some facilities could have an array of different machines that help during the preparation process, such as pumps. Pumps are devices used to "pump" fluids from one container to another. They help reduce manipulations and secure accurate quantities.

When working with equipment such as this, it is extremely important that personnel receive proper training and/or education to be competent in using these machines. Remember that even though the equipment may seem automated, it generally still requires input from personnel to calibrate or request functions. And because many of these devices rely on software functions, it can be easy to put the wrong information in the wrong places; some systems produce flags or warnings that pop up like computer error messages when something has been entered incorrectly. Also, remember that a pharmacist supervises the process and will be checking off the final product. Many procedures require that a pharmacist check after setting up the equipment and before the actual adding or pumping takes place.

Here are some examples of pumps you may see:

- **Automix** An automated device used to compound TPN bases.
- **Micromix** An automated device used to add additives to a TPN base.

CONCLUSION

As with any professional skill, specific equipment and supplies are required to properly prepare sterile products. When using aseptic technique, you must also follow stringent guidelines pertaining to the facility and appropriate dress. Thorough knowledge and understanding of each of the facilities, equipment, and garb detailed in this chapter should be acquired prior to practical, hands-on experience.

PROFILES OF PRACTICE

One of the topics addressed by USP 797 is personnel training and evaluation. Several states require pharmacy technicians to be certified in sterile product preparation and aseptic technique in order to work in the clean room environment. Requirements vary from state to state, but can include as many as 40 hr of ACPE-accredited continuing education focused on aseptic technique with 20 hr of validated, practical experience.

A number of employers, colleges, and national organizations offer sterile product certification courses for pharmacy technicians, including a national certification course offered by the National Pharmacy Technician Association (NPTA).

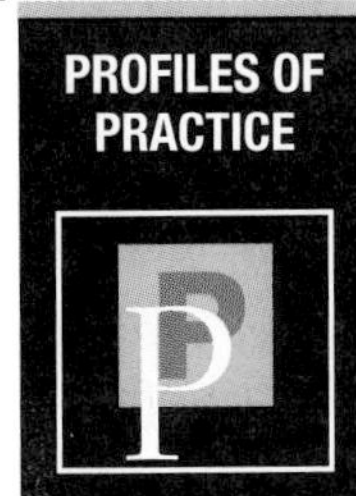

CHAPTER TERMS

anteroom
the room located right outside the clean room; it is a low-particulate room, which means that it should not contain paper, boxes, or high-particulate matter. Food and drink should not be allowed in this room

desiccation
the act of dehydrating or removing water content

germicidal
describes an agent that kills pathogenic microorganisms

particulates
small matter

single dose vial (SDV)
a vial that contains no preservatives, once the container is entered, contaminants may have been introduced and the container is no longer sterile

vial
a small bottle or container that holds products such as injectable medications

CHAPTER 2

CHAPTER REVIEW QUESTIONS

MULTIPLE CHOICE

1. All of the following materials belong in an anteroom except __________.
   a. shoe covers
   b. gowning material
   c. cardboard boxes
   d. sticky mats
   e. antimicrobial soap

2. Which of the following materials do not belong in a clean room? __________
   a. laminar airflow hood
   b. biological safety cabinet
   c. paper towels
   d. 70% isopropyl alcohol
   e. stainless steel cart

3. A full hand washing should be done __________.
   a. upon entry into the clean area
   b. after eating lunch or a snack
   c. after a restroom break
   d. only a and c
   e. a, b, and c

4. What materials are needed to perform a full hood cleaning? __________
   a. sterile water, 70% isopropyl alcohol, lint-free paper towels/gauze
   b. tap water, 70% isopropyl alcohol, paper towels
   c. sterile water, 90% isopropyl alcohol, lint-free paper towels
   d. sterile water, 70% isopropyl alcohol, paper towels
   e. paper towels, 70% isopropyl alcohol, antimicrobial soap

5. The direction of airflow in a biological safety cabinet is __________.
   a. horizontal from back to front
   b. horizontal from front to back
   c. vertical from top to bottom
   d. vertical from bottom to top
   e. horizontal from left to right

6. A filter needle is primarily used for removing __________.
   a. bubbles from a syringe
   b. glass shards and other particulates from a solution
   c. virons and bacteria from a solution
   d. all of the above
   e. a and c only

7. __________ are used for transferring the contents of one syringe to another.
   a. Viaflex bags
   b. dispensing pins
   c. leur-to-leur connectors
   d. filter needles/filter straws
   e. metric cylinders

8. __________, which are a needleless system, are used to remove the contents of a vial into a syringe.

a. Viaflex bags
b. Dispensing pins
c. Leur-to-leur connectors
d. Filter needles/filter straws
e. Leur-lock connectors

9. __________ are empty plastic IV bags that are used as an empty, sterile container.

a. Viaflex bags
b. Dispensing pins
c. Leur-to-leur connectors
d. Empty evacuated containers
e. Vacuums

10. The LAH must be turned on for at least __________ before any aseptic compounding can take place.

a. 30 min
b. 15 min
c. 1 hr
d. 24 hr
e. 20 min

11. How often should the prefilter be changed? __________

a. yearly
b. quarterly
c. monthly
d. weekly
e. biweekly

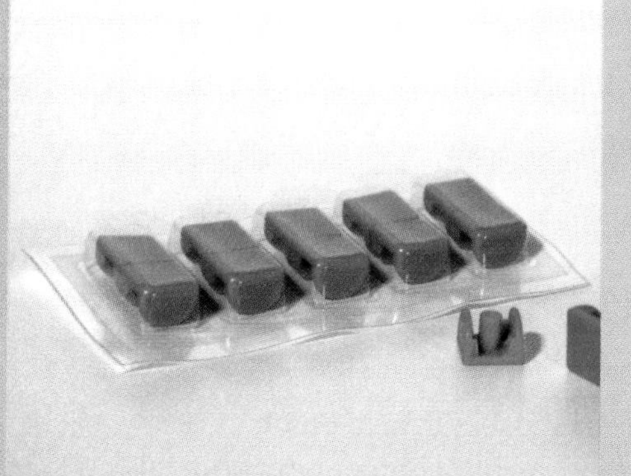

CHAPTER 3

Aseptic Calculations

Learning Objectives

After completing this chapter, you should be able to:

- Show calculations related to products prepared using aseptic technique.
- Calculate the quantity of active ingredient needed for each preparation.
- Calculate the volume of active ingredient to add to an IV admixture.
- Calculate the volume of electrolytes to add to a TPN.
- Determine the rate of flow for IV meds.
- Discuss and calculate dilution technique.

INTRODUCTION

For the purposes of this chapter, it is assumed that you have already mastered basic calculations skills; if you have not mastered basic pharmacy calculations, please refer to *The Pharmacy Technician Series—Pharmacy Calculations*, published by Prentice Hall Health. While the use of aseptic technique is necessary when preparing products in the clean room, the calculations that are required are equally important to ensure product integrity and patient safety.

Active Ingredient

To determine the amount of active ingredient needed to make a preparation, multiply the milligrams of active ingredient per milliliter by the number of milliliters to be prepared. Use ratios and proportions and cross-multiply when appropriate.

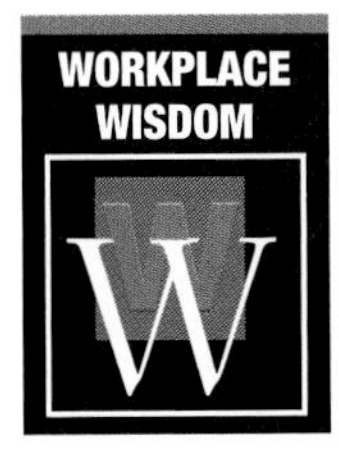

Powders weighed on an electronic balance are weighed in grams; therefore, milligrams are converted to grams.

EXAMPLE 3.1 Rx hydroxycobalamine 5000 mcg/mL 30 mL

How many grams of active ingredient should you weigh out?

Convert micrograms to milligrams by moving the decimal three places to the left: 5000 mcg is the same as 5 mg.

$$5 \text{ mg} \times 30 \text{ mL} = 150 \text{ mg}$$

Convert milligrams to grams by moving the decimal three places to the left: 150 mg is the same as 0.15 g.

EXAMPLE 3.2 Rx taurine 50 mg/mL 45 mL

How many grams of active ingredient should you weigh out?

$$50 \text{ mg} \times 45 \text{ mL} = 2250 \text{ mg}$$

Convert milligrams to grams by moving the decimal three places to the left: 2250 mg is the same as 2.25 g.

IV Admixtures

Many preparations prepared in the clean room are considered IV admixtures. IV bags generally contain either normal saline (NS) or dextrose 5% in water (D5W). The contents of IV bags are sterile. Active ingredients such as antibiotics, vitamins, and electrolytes are added using the principles of aseptic technique. Calculating the volume of active ingredient to be added is critical. Incidental amounts are added to the volume of the IV bag. When adding a larger volume, you must withdraw an equal volume from the IV bag before adding the active ingredient. IV bags have an injection port for this process.

EXAMPLE 3.3 Rx vancomycin 500 mg/250 mL

What is the concentration of the IV preparation?

$$\frac{500 \text{ mg}}{250 \text{ mL}} = \frac{x \text{ mg}}{1 \text{ mL}}$$

$$250x = 500$$

$$x = 2 \text{ mg/mL}$$

Vancomycin powder for injection is available in a variety of sizes, such as 500-mg vials, 1-g vials, 5-g vials, and 10-g vials. Instructions on each stock vial indicate how many milliliters of sterile water for injection you should add for reconstitution.

In addition, the manufacturer notes that a number of compatible IV diluents can be used, including 5% dextrose, 0.9% saline, or lactated Ringer's, which is a combined solution of electrolytes. Administration should last at least 60 min.

To reconstitute the 500-mg vial of powder for injection, add 10 mL of sterile water for injection. This will then be injected into a 250-mL bag of 0.9% saline for injection.

EXAMPLE 3.4 Rx levofloxacin 750 mg qs to yield 5 mg/mL in D5W

How many milliliters of IV diluent will you need to yield 5 mg/mL?

$$\frac{750\text{ mg}}{x} = \frac{5\text{ mg}}{1\text{ mL}}$$
$$5x = 750$$
$$x = 150\text{ mL}$$

Levofloxacin is available in concentrates of 500 mg and 750 mg per vial premixed with sterile water for injection, both at a concentration of 25 mg/mL. How many milliliters are in the 500-mg vial?

$$\frac{500\text{ mg}}{x} = \frac{25\text{ mg}}{1\text{ mL}}$$
$$25x = 500$$
$$x = 20\text{ mL}$$

How many milliliters are in the 750-mg vial?

$$\frac{750\text{ mg}}{x} = \frac{25\text{ mg}}{1\text{ mL}}$$
$$25x = 750$$
$$x = 30\text{ mL}$$

The concentrate will be diluted into a compatible IV diluent such as 0.9% saline or D5W. The IV should be administered slowly over 60–90 min and given every 24 hr as indicated by the infection.

Flow Rates

Once an IV admixture is prepared, it is delivered to the patient and set up using an administration set. The mini-drip administration set delivers 60 drops per milliliter. Unless noted, always assume 60 gtt./mL when setting up the formula for calculating flow rates. If you are using an administration set that is calibrated differently, it will be noted, and then you should insert the new information into the formula.

WORKPLACE WISDOM

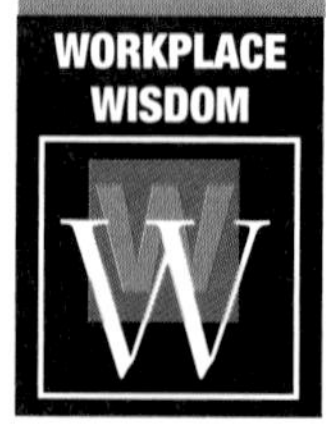

When using dimensional analysis, assume 60 gtt./1 mL unless otherwise noted in the problem.

Dimensional analysis is a method of setting up the flow rate formula that enables you to solve the problem efficiently by using logical sequencing and placing units so that you can cancel them out to leave the desired terms for the answer.

The formula, using dimensional analysis, is as follows:

$$\frac{\text{mL}}{\text{hr}} \times \frac{\text{gtt.}}{1\text{ mL}} \times \frac{1\text{ hr}}{60\text{ min}} = \text{gtt./min}$$

EXAMPLE 3.5 Rx vancomycin 500 mg/250 mL over 120 min

Determine the flow rate in gtt./min.

$$\frac{250 \text{ mL}}{2 \text{ hr}} \times \frac{60 \text{ gtt.}}{1 \text{ mL}} \times \frac{1 \text{ hr}}{60 \text{ min}} = 125 \text{ gtt./min}$$

EXAMPLE 3.6 Rx levofloxacin 750 mg qs to yield 5 mg/mL over 90 min

Determine the flow rate in mL/hr.

Determine how many milliliters are required to maintain the concentration of 5 mg/mL:

$$\frac{5 \text{ mg}}{1 \text{ mL}} :: \frac{750 \text{ mg}}{x \text{ mL}} = 150 \text{ mL}$$

Divide by the total administration time to determine the rate:

$$\frac{150 \text{ mL}}{1.5 \text{ hr}} = 100 \text{ mL/hr}$$

Electrolytes Added to Total Parenteral Nutrition (TPN) Preparations

Electrolytes are charged ions in solution that are important in maintaining acid-base balance in body fluids, controlling body water volume, and regulating metabolism. Milliequivalents are used to express the concentration of electrolytes in solution.

Electrolyte solutions and TPNs are administered intravenously. TPN is used when the patient cannot consume food or nutritional formula orally. TPNs contain a balanced emulsion of sugar, protein, fats, minerals, electrolytes, vitamins, and water. Many TPNs are called 3-in-1 solutions because they contain fats, amino acids, and dextrose. These should be injected into the IV bag in the order "FAD": fats, then amino acids, then dextrose. Once this base emulsion is made, the electrolytes are added last before labeling.

Electrolytes are available in stock vials with the concentration noted on the vial. To determine the volume needed, simply note the total milliequivalents of ingredient required and divide by the concentration noted on the vial.

EXAMPLE 3.7 Determine the volume needed for each of the following electrolytes.

NaCl

Stock vial concentration = 4 mEq/mL
Milliequivalents ordered = 60 mEq
Volume needed: 60 mEq/4 mEq = 15 mL

Na phosphate

Stock vial concentration = 4 mEq/mL
Milliequivalents ordered = 40 mEq
Volume needed: 40 mEq/4 mEq = 10 mL

K acetate

Stock vial concentration = 2 mEq/mL

Milliequivalents ordered = 24 mEq
Volume needed: 24 mEq/2 mEq = 12 mL

$MgSO_4$

Stock vial concentration = 4 mEq/mL
Milliequivalents ordered = 35 mEq
Volume needed: 35 mEq/4 mEq = 8.75 mL

Na acetate

Stock vial concentration = 2 mEq/mL
Milliequivalents ordered = 12 mEq
Volume needed: 12 mEq/2 mEq = 6 mL

KCl

Stock vial concentration = 2 mEq/mL
Milliequivalents ordered = 42 mEq
Volume needed: 42 mEq/2 mEq = 21 mL

K phosphate

Stock vial concentration = 4.4 mEq/mL
Milliequivalents ordered = 13 mEq
Volume needed: 13 mEq/4.4 mEq = 2.95 mL

Ca gluconate

Stock vial concentration = 0.465 mEq/mL
Milliequivalents ordered = 20 mEq
Volume needed: 20 mEq/0.465 mEq = 43.01 mL

TPNs contain a number of electrolytes that start out in a stock vial. The milliliters required are drawn into a syringe and injected into a TPN bag through the injection port and prepared for IV administration. After calculating the volume of each component needed for the order, add them up to determine the total volume of electrolytes. In Example 3.7, the total volume of electrolytes, from Na phosphate to Ca gluconate, is 103.7 mL.

Dilution Technique

A few medications have such a minute dosage that dilution is required. The general procedure for diluting is to dilute 1 mL of the concentrate with 9 mL of sterile water for injection. Then take 1 mL of that concentration and further dilute it with 9 mL of sterile water for injection. To further dilute, take 1 mL of that concentration and dilute it with 9 mL of sterile water for injection, and so on. A new empty sterile vial is utilized for each subsequent dilution.

EXAMPLE 3.8 Rx insulin dilution to 10 U/mL

Take 1 mL from a stock vial containing 100 U/mL and inject it into an empty sterile vial. Add 9 mL of sterile water for injection. What is the resulting concentration?

Answer: 100 U/10 mL or 10 U/1 mL

If a patient requires a dose of three units once daily, what volume should be injected?

$$\frac{10\text{ U}}{1\text{ mL}} :: \frac{3\text{ U}}{x\text{ mL}} = 0.3\text{ mL}$$

Pediatric Formulas

Children need lower dosages of medication compared to adults. There are three formulas to help you calculate a pediatric dosage based on whatever information is available. You must know a child's weight in order to calculate a medication dosage. Most pediatric doses are based on body weight in kilograms. In some children's hospitals the pharmacy may have a preferred formula; however, the pharmacy technician should be able to calculate the correct pediatric dosage using each formula:

Fried's Rule

$$\text{Child's dosage} = \frac{\text{Age in months}}{150} \times \text{Adult dosage}$$

Young's Rule

$$\text{Child's dosage} = \frac{\text{Age of child in years}}{\text{Age of child in years} + 12} \times \text{Adult dosage}$$

Clark's Rule

$$\text{Child's dosage} = \frac{\text{Child's weight in pounds}}{150} \times \text{Adult dosage}$$

EXAMPLE 3.9 A 1-year-old child weighs approximately 16 lb. The normal adult dosage is 800 mg. What is the child's dose using each formula?

Fried's Rule

$$x = \frac{12\text{ months}}{150} \times 800$$
$$= 64\text{ mg}$$

Young's Rule

$$x = \frac{1}{1 + 12} \times 800$$
$$= 61.5\text{ mg}$$

Clark's Rule

$$x = \frac{16}{150} \times 800$$
$$= 85\text{ mg}$$

Body Surface Area and Nomograms

Not all dosing calculations are based strictly on body weight. *Body surface area (BSA)* is used to determine dosages that are based on the patient's height and weight. Medications that have wide therapeutic ranges and short durations of action can be calculated on body weight alone. But the BSA is generally calculated and used for dosing agents with narrow therapeutic indices, such as those for pediatric dosing, radiation and oncologic therapy, amputees, severe burn patients, renal disease, and open-heart surgery.

The major advantages of calculating dosages based on the BSA are as follows:

1. BSA provides a more accurate cross-species comparison of activity and toxicity for certain drugs.
2. BSA can be more closely correlated with cardiac output, which determines the blood flow to the liver and kidneys, thus influencing drug elimination.

Due to the importance of exact dosing for patient safety, antineoplastic and highly potent drugs are always calculated using the BSA. BSA should be recalculated when body weight has changed by greater than 5–10 percent.

BSA can be calculated by a formula or by use of a chart called a *nomogram*. Several formulas that have been developed are shown here, with the Mosteller being the most popular and widely used.

- Formula of Mosteller (adults and children)[1]:

$$\text{BSA (m}^2\text{)} = \sqrt{\frac{\text{Height (cm)} \times \text{Weight (kg)}}{3600}} \text{ or } \sqrt{\frac{\text{Height (in.)} \times \text{Weight (lb.)}}{3131}}$$

  This formula is a simple modification of an equation by Gehan and George and requires the use of a calculator with a square root key. The formula has been confirmed as being applicable to children by Lam and Leung.

- Formula of Gehan and George[2]:

  $$\text{BSA (m}^2\text{)} = \text{Weight (kg)}^{0.51456} \times \text{Height (cm)}^{0.42246} \times 0.02350$$

- Formula of DuBois and DuBois[3]:

  $$\text{BSA (m}^2\text{)} = \text{Weight (kg)}^{0.425} \times \text{Height (cm)}^{0.725} \times 0.007184$$

  This is the classic formula, published in 1916, on which many nomograms are based.

- Formula of Haycock et al.[4]:

  $$\text{BSA (m}^2\text{)} = \text{Weight (kg)}^{0.5378} \times \text{Height (cm)}^{0.3964} \times 0.024265$$

To estimate an adult's BSA with the following nomogram (Figure 3-1), use a straightedge to connect the patient's weight in the right column with his height in the left column. The point of intersection in the middle column is the BSA. For example, a patient who weighs 120 lb. and is 62 in. tall has a BSA of 1.60 m^2.

[1] R. D. Mosteller. "Simplified Calculation of Body-Surface Area." *New England Journal of Medicine* 317 (1987): 1098.

[2] E. A. Gehan and S. L. George. "Estimation of Human Body Surface Area from Height and Weight." *Cancer Chemotherapy Report* 54 (1970): 225–235.

[3] D. DuBois and D. F. DuBois. "A Formula to Estimate the Approximate Surface Area If Height and Weight Be Known." *Archives of Intenal Medicine* 17 (1916): 863–871.

[4] G. B. Haycock, G. J. Schwartz, and D. H. Wisotsky. "Geometric Method for Measuring Body Surface Area: A Height-Weight Formula Validated in Infants, Children and Adults." *Journal of Pediatrics* 93 (1978): 62–66.

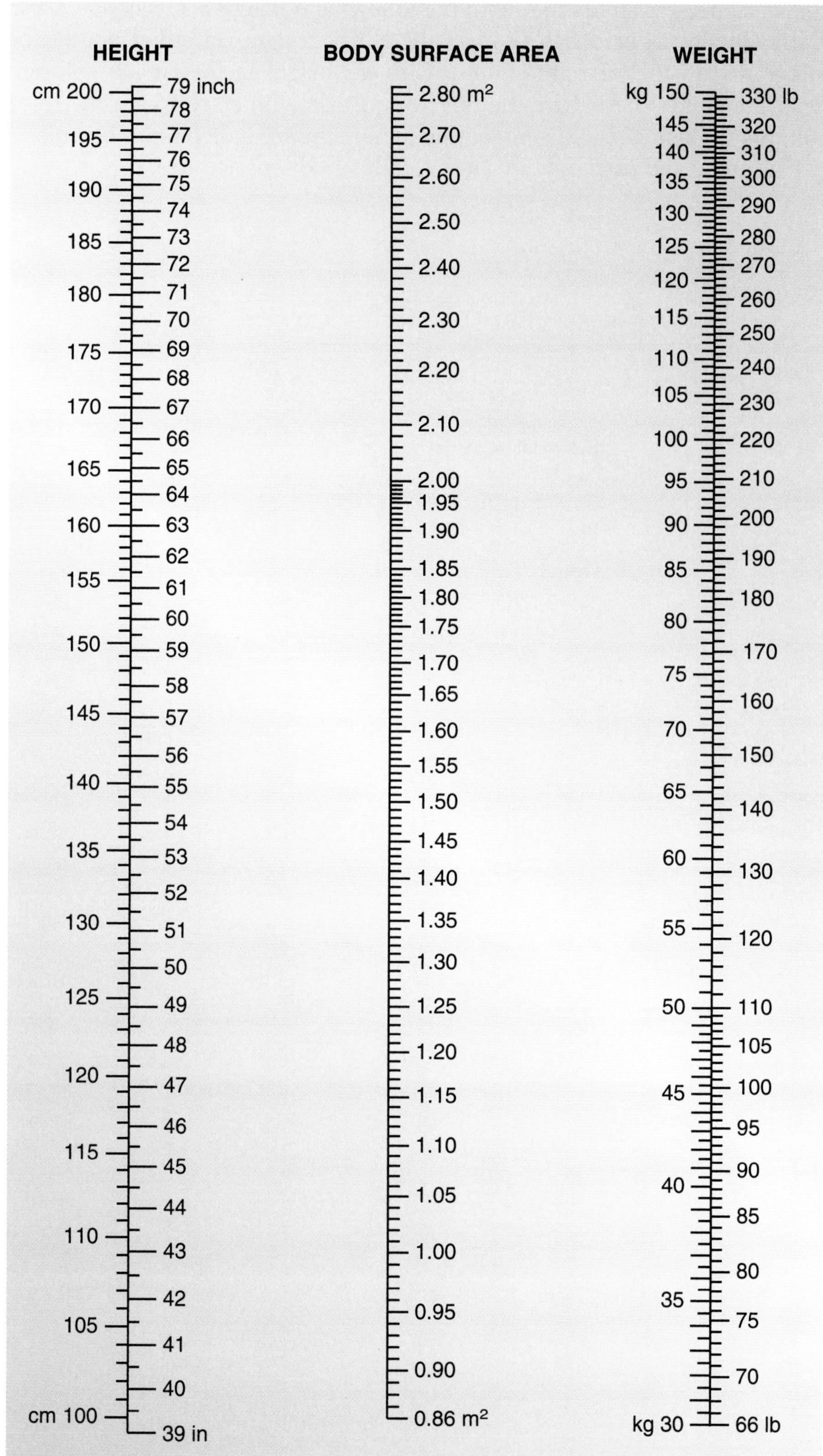

Figure 3-1 Adult nomogram

To estimate a child's BSA with the following nomogram (Figure 3-2), use a straightedge as before to connect the child's weight (in either pounds or kilograms) in the far right column with his height in the far left column. Read the child's BSA where the line you just drew intersects with the third column. (When using this nomogram, ignore the second column. It is mostly inaccurate and used only to guess a child's body surface area.)

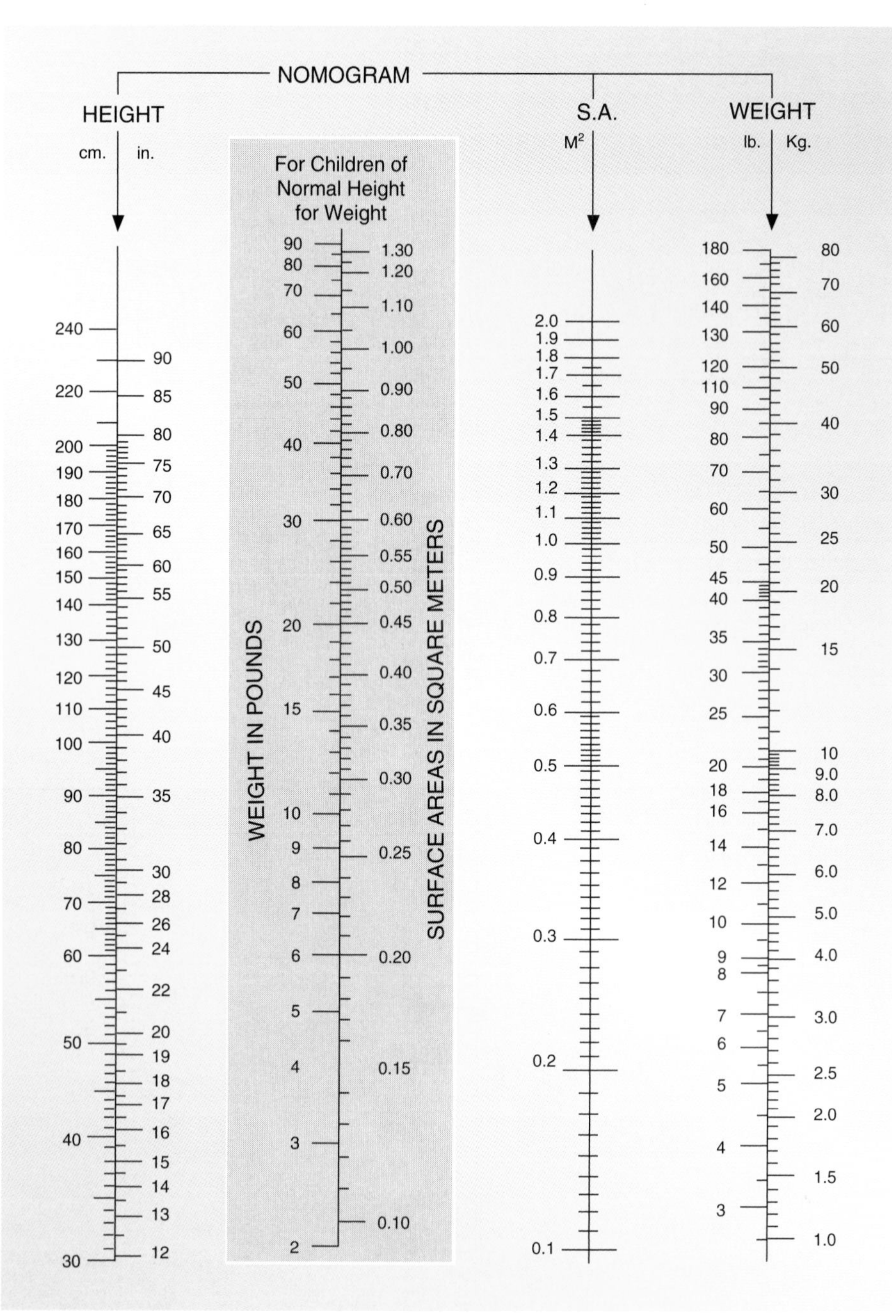

Figure 3-2 Child nomogram

Dosage Calculations

This is an example of a simple straightforward proportion. A competent IV technician is extremely proficient with these calculations.

EXAMPLE 3.10 What is the concentration of a 1-g vancomycin vial that is reconstituted with 20 mL of water?

Make any necessary conversions (most concentrations are measured in mg/mL): 1 g = 1000 mg

$$\frac{1000 \text{ mg}}{20 \text{ mL}} = \frac{x \text{ mg}}{1 \text{ mL}}$$

Cross-multiply and solve for x:

$$20x = 1000$$
$$x = 50 \text{ mg/mL}$$

EXAMPLE 3.11 A physician orders a grasshopper solution for an emergency room patient. On his order he specifies that he wants at least 50 mL of the grasshopper solution. The grasshopper solution contains 25 mg/5 mL of diphenhydramine. How much diphenhydramine will be in 50 mL?

Make sure to set up the proportion correctly. The numerators should have the same label. The denominators should also have the same label:

$$\frac{25 \text{ mg}}{5 \text{ mL}} = \frac{x \text{ mg}}{50 \text{ mL}}$$

Cross-multiply and solve for x:

$$1250 = 5x$$
$$x = 250 \text{ mg}$$

EXAMPLE 3.12 A physician orders tobramycin 150 mg in D5W IVPB. If tobramycin comes as 40 mg/mL, how many milliliters should be added to the D5W IVPB?

Make sure to set up the proportion correctly. The numerators should have the same units. The denominators should also have the same units:

$$\frac{40 \text{ mg}}{1 \text{ mL}} = \frac{150 \text{ mg}}{x \text{ mL}}$$

Cross-multiply and solve for x:

$$40x = 150$$
$$x = 3.75 \text{ mL}$$

EXAMPLE 3.13 A physician orders a pediatric syringe that should contain 450 mg of an antibiotic called Claforan. If Claforan comes as 1000 mg/10 mL, how many milliliters will you need for the correct dose?

Make sure to set up the proportion correctly. The numerators should have the same units. The denominators should also have the same units:

$$\frac{1000 \text{ mg}}{10 \text{ mL}} = \frac{450 \text{ mg}}{x \text{ mL}}$$

Cross-multiply and solve for x:

$$1000x = 4500$$
$$x = 4.5 \text{ mL of Claforan}$$

PRACTICE PROBLEMS 3.1

1. Rx testosterone cypionate 100 mg/mL 10 mL
   How many grams of active ingredient should you weigh out? ___________
2. Rx testosterone enanthate 200 mg/mL 5 mL
   How many grams of active ingredient should you weigh out? ___________
3. Rx dexamethasone sodium phosphate 4 mg/mL 30 mL
   How many grams of active ingredient should you weigh out? ___________
4. Rx cefuroxime 2 g powder for injection

   Add 19.2 mL diluent (2 g/20 mL)

   75 mg/kg/day divided q12h

   Patient weighs 44 lb.

   1 kg = 2.2 lb.

   How many milliliters of active ingredient should you inject into the IV bag? ________________
5. Rx furosemide 80 mg at 4 mg/min
   How many minutes will it take to administer the furosemide? ___________
6. Rx phenytoin 50 mg/mL

   5 mg/kg

   Patient weighs 132 lb.

   1 kg = 2.2 lb.

   How many milliliters of active ingredient should you inject directly into the IV line? ________________
7. Rx D5W 1000 mL over 12 hr
   What is the flow rate in gtt./min? ________________
8. Rx cefuroxime 750 mg/100 mL over 30 min q8h
   What is the flow rate in gtt./min? ________________
9. Rx TPN with electrolytes
   How many milliliters of each of the following electrolytes should you inject into the TPN bag? ________________

   a. NaCl

      Stock vial concentration = 4 mEq/mL

      Milliequivalents ordered = 24 mEq

      Volume needed: ________________

b. **Na phosphate**
   Stock vial concentration = 4 mEq/mL
   Milliequivalents ordered = 24 mEq
   Volume needed: ________________

c. **K acetate**
   Stock vial concentration = 2 mEq/mL
   Milliequivalents ordered = 12 mEq
   Volume needed: ________________

d. **$MgSO_4$**
   Stock vial concentration = 4 mEq/mL
   Milliequivalents ordered = 40 mEq
   Volume needed: ________________

e. **Na acetate**
   Stock vial concentration = 2 mEq/mL
   Milliequivalents ordered = 10 mEq
   Volume needed: ________________

f. **KCl**
   Stock vial concentration = 2 mEq/mL
   Milliequivalents ordered = 38 mEq
   Volume needed: ________________

g. **K phosphate**
   Stock vial concentration = 4.4 mEq/mL
   Milliequivalents ordered = 22 mEq
   Volume needed: ________________

h. **Ca gluconate**
   Stock vial concentration = 0.465 mEq/mL
   Milliequivalents ordered = 18 mEq
   Volume needed: ________________

i. What is the total volume of electrolytes to be added:

   ____

10. Rx prostaglandin-E 10 mcg/mL
    If the stock container of prostaglandin-E is 100 mg/mL, how many 9-mL dilutions are required? ________________

CONCLUSION

Clearly, many calculations are required when working with sterile products; this chapter has covered the most common calculations a pharmacy technician will encounter in this setting, but it cannot replace a strong comprehension of all pharmacy calculations. Many aseptic calculations seem overwhelming and intimidating at first glance; however, nearly all are solved using simple algebraic principles or ratios/proportions.

CHAPTER REVIEW QUESTIONS

MULTIPLE CHOICE

Rx penicillin G potassium
250,000 U/kg/day up to 20,000 U/day
Patient weighs 160 lb.
IV administered over 24 hr
20,000,000 U/L
1 kg = 2.2 lb.

1. What is the patient's weight in kilograms? __________
   a. 308 kg
   b. 63.63 kg
   c. 72.73 kg
   d. 80 kg
   e. 22.2 kg

2. How many units of penicillin G potassium are needed for one day? __________
   a. 18,182,500 U/day
   b. 3437 U/day
   c. 1562 U/day
   d. 20,000,000 U/day
   e. 5,000,000 U/day

3. How many milliliters will you need to extract from the 20,000,000 U/L IV bag of penicillin G potassium and what will be the resultant volume? __________
   a. 30 mL, 970 mL
   b. 60 mL, 940 mL
   c. 91 mL, 909 mL
   d. 81 mL, 923 mL
   e. 101 mL, 899 mL

4. What is the flow rate of the penicillin G potassium in mL/hr? __________
   a. 30 mL/hr
   b. 25 mL/hr
   c. 38 mL/hr
   d. 42 mL/hr
   e. 14 mL/hr

5. How many units/minute of penicillin G potassium will the patient receive? __________
   a. 10,500 U/min
   b. 12,560 U/min
   c. 12,602 U/min
   d. 13,000 U/min
   e. 10,200 U/min

Rx dexamethasone sodium phosphate
0.25 mg/kg/dose q8h
Patient weighs 44 lb.
Dose is administered over 30 min
Stock vial 4 mg/mL in 10-mL vials
50-mL IV bag
IV administration set delivers 20 gtt./mL

6. What is the patient's weight in kilograms? __________
   a. 10 kg
   b. 20 kg
   c. 88 kg
   d. 33 kg
   e. 44 kg

7. What is the dose in milligrams of dexamethasone sodium phosphate? __________
   a. 1.67 mg
   b. 2.5 mg
   c. 4.4 mg
   d. 5.0 mg
   e. 2.0 mg

8. What is the daily dose in grams of dexamethasone sodium phosphate? __________
   a. 0.015 g
   b. 0.050 g
   c. 1.0 g
   d. 15 g
   e. 0.051 g

9. How many milliliters of dexamethasone sodium phosphate will you need from the stock vial? __________
   a. 0.4 mL
   b. 1.0 mL
   c. 1.25 mL
   d. 1.15 mL
   e. 1.5 mL

10. What is the flow rate of the dexamethasone sodium phosphate in gtt./min? __________
   a. 100 gtt./min
   b. 44 gtt./min
   c. 15 gtt./min
   d. 33 gtt./min
   e. 22 gtt./min

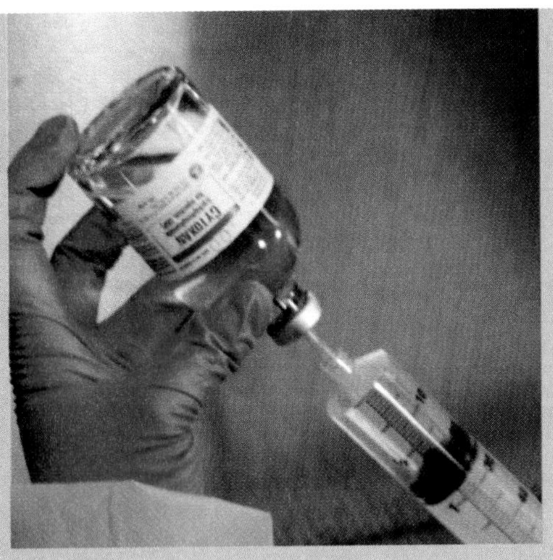

CHAPTER 4

Properties of Sterile Products

Learning Objectives

After completing this chapter, you should be able to:

- Explain the cautions associated with microbial contamination.
- Understand the pH range and why it is important.
- Understand the concepts of compatibility and stability.
- Explain the difference between tonicity, osmolarity, and osmolality.
- Know how to calculate the osmolarity of an IV solution.

INTRODUCTION

Sterile products may be compounded for use as inhalants, enterals, topicals, ophthalmics and otics. The primary focus of this textbook, however, is on IV aseptic preparations and technique. The fundamental knowledge you acquire will apply to all sterile preparations made for the previously mentioned administrations. We will focus on IVs, as this is the most common parenteral method used today.

We cannot emphasize enough the importance of preparing a product that is free from particulates, pyrogens, and other contaminants. Injectables are administered in such a way that they bypass one of the greatest barriers to contamination—the skin. Because of this increased risk, it is extremely important that the pharmacy technician who is preparing a sterile product understand the consequences of poor technique and dangers to the patient who receives the medication.

The finished sterile product should be free of contamination. The solutions should also be clear and all medications should be completely dissolved. Keep in mind that some ingredients may be somewhat darker, but there should not be anything floating around in the final product that does not belong—for example, matter that has entered from the outside or that forms a solid as a chemical reaction between the ingredients.

Compounders who prepare sterile products must be fully aware of some considerations. We will discuss some of the most important topics in this chapter.

Particulate Matter

While preparing a product that requires transferring the ingredients of one container to another, be very careful not to allow any portion of the package to transfer along with the medication. For example, when drawing up from a vial with the typical rubber top, if you do not insert the needle correctly, you may unknowingly enter the rubber stopper with the needle and transfer small portions of the rubber into the base solution bag. This is known as **coring**. Other undissolved substances of great concern are glass, cloth, plastic, metals, and other substances. Such particulate matter injected into the vein can lodge and block blood flow or cause inflammation and possible infection (sepsis), as a foreign matter has invaded the body. Be certain to visually inspect every product you prepare for "floaties" or other unusual differences that should not be present, regardless of how many times you make a product (Figure 4–1).

coring
transferring part of the rubber stopper of a vial or container into a solution bag because of improper needle stick

WORKPLACE WISDOM

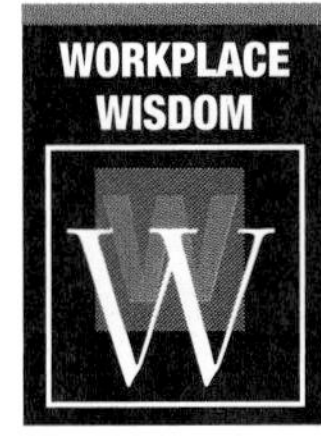

Do not take anything for granted or become comfortable enough to hot perform a visual check. The pharmacist signing off on this final product will expect you have done this and will be looking for the same as an additional safety precaution and as part of the multiple check procedure.

pH, Acids, and Bases

pH refers to a measure of how acidic or basic a solution is. The *p* stands for *potenz*, meaning "potential to be," and the *H* is for *hydrogen*. The pH scale ranges from 0 (extremely acidic) to 14 (extremely basic). In the middle of this scale is pure water at 7.0 (neutral). A neutral solution is neither too **acidic** nor too **alkaline** (basic). With few exceptions, life exists in a fairly narrow range of pH. Therefore, pH is considerably important in understanding normal cellular functions and values as well as the relationship between acids and bases.

Bases are substances that increase the number of hydroxide ions (OH^-), and thus remove hydrogen ions. By reducing the concentration of hydrogen atoms, bases raise the pH. So as the H^+ concentration increases, the pH decreases. The more H^+ in solution, the more acidic the solution becomes and the lower the pH falls. As the H^+ concentration increases, the pH decreases, thus becoming more acidic (Figure 4–1).

acidic
describes a substance that increases the concentration of hydrogen ions (lowers the pH); an acidic substance is called an acid

alkaline
describes a substance that decreases the concentration of hydrogen ions (raises the pH); an alkaline substance is called a base

THE PH SCALE

The pH scale is logarithmic; a decrease of one unit on this scale represents multiplying acidity ten times. For example, bleach is 10 times as basic as soapy water. Acid rain is 100 times as acidic as urine. A pH of 6.9 or below is considered an acid; anything 7.1 and above is considered an alkali or base.

The pH of a solution is important as it could affect how products react together. When a product reacts, it can cause precipitation, heat, gas, or cloudiness. As medications are considered chemicals, mixing certain drugs together can change the pH of a solution, sometimes making them

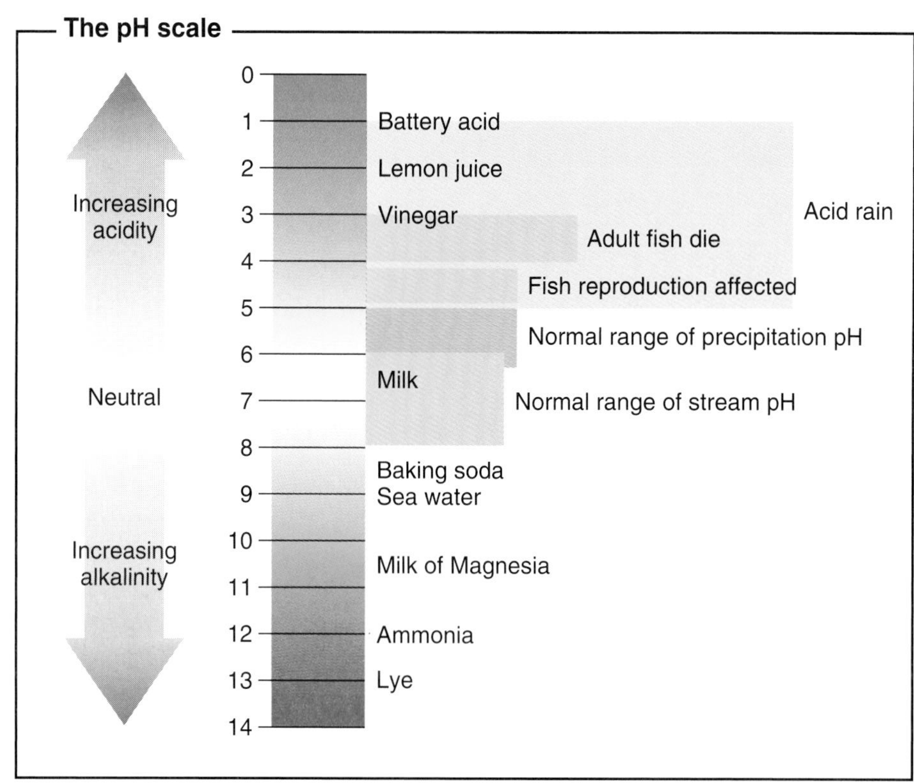

Figure 4-1 pH scale

incompatible. When a solution becomes incompatible, precipitation or crystallization can occur.

Human blood is pH 7.4 (blood plasma needs slightly alkaline, or slightly salty, pH). Most parenteral solutions are slightly acidic, in the pH range of 3.5 to 6.2. For example, dextrose 5% is slightly more acidic than human blood and therefore can sometimes sting a little while being infused. Think of it like this: Ordinary bar soap has a slightly lower pH than that of the human eye. So when it gets in your eyes, it stings! Chemical reactions in the body are very sensitive to even slight changes in the acidity or alkalinity of the body fluids in which they occur. Any departure from the narrow limits of normal H^+ and OH^- concentrations greatly disrupts body functions.

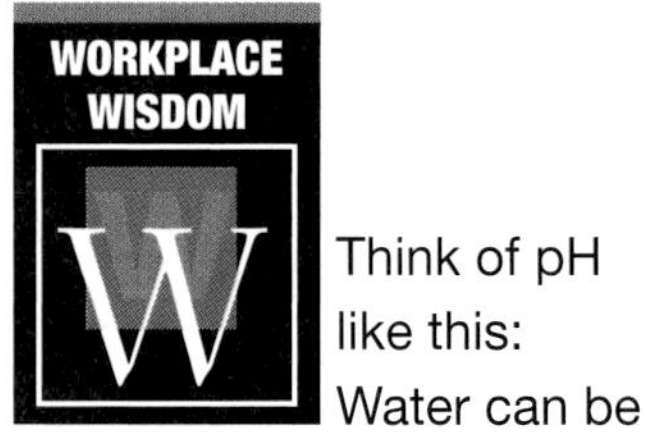

Think of pH like this: Water can be hot or cold; these extremes of temperature can be neutralized by mixing hot and cold, to even out the temperature. The same theory applies with acids and bases. You can add one or the other to adjust the pH balance.

Compatibility and Stability

Like pH, compatibility is an extremely important factor in preparations. As mentioned, sometimes incompatibility can result in precipitation or crystallization, but sometimes incompatibility is not always visible. Added drugs can interact with each other, enhance one another, or even cancel each other out.

Basically, there are three major types of incompatibilities: physical, chemical, and therapeutic.

- **Physical**—This is the easiest incompatibility to identify, as it results in a physical change to the product such as precipitation, cloudiness, hot or cold presence while mixing, change in color, or separation.

It is usually caused by a chemical reaction or when ingredients do not mix.

- **Chemical**—Chemical incompatibility occurs when a chemical reaction causes a change in the molecular structure or activity of the ingredients.
- **Therapeutic**—Therapeutic incompatibility occurs when giving two or more drugs within a short period of time results in decreased effectiveness of one or more of the ingredients.

As a pharmacy technician involved with sterile compounding, you will become familiar with compatibility through extensive experience and with the help of available literature resources such as *Trissel's Handbook of Injectable Drugs*, one of the most widely used references available today. *Trissel's* contains detailed compatibility and stability information for many injectable solutions. Other factors to consider with incompatibility include concentrations and dilutions of the product, the order of mixing, and preservatives that may be added.

It is important to note that not all reactions due to incompatibilities appear right away and may even take hours to become visible. All incompatibilities affect the stability of a preparation. However, stability considerations are typically broader and include the overall assurance that the integrity of the formulation is maintained until the product is administered to a patient.

Each product, once made, has an expiration date. Stability refers to the ability of the product to remain stable until used or until the expiration date is reached. Many factors contribute to stability such as temperature, length of time on shelf before use, light sensitivity, or chemical reactions over time including reduced effectiveness.

In a hospital-type setting, sterile compounded products typically maintain an average shelf life of 24–48 hr, as they are constantly made at determined intervals, sometimes around the clock. For other situations, such as long-term or home care, the typical shelf life is around 30 days. As you may read in references such as *Trissel's*, refrigerating or freezing some products often extends the shelf life. However, some preparations cannot be stored under refrigeration as it would negatively affect the stability and/or compatibility. The key is to understand that each product requires a certain set of instructions regarding preparation and storage. As a professional pharmacy technician, you must be able to research and understand these requirements.

Tonicity

The tonicity of an IV fluid dictates whether the solution should be administered by the peripheral or central venous route. Hypotonic and hypertonic solutions may be infused in small volumes and into large vessels, where dilution and distribution are rapid. If a solution varies greatly from the normal range, it may cause tissue irritation, pain on injection, or electrolyte shifts.

Tonicity refers to the response of cells or tissues to the solutions in which they are immersed. Picture a membrane separating two solutions, one side with a higher solute concentration than the other.

- The side with the higher solute concentration is hypertonic.
- The side with the lower solute concentration is hypotonic.
- If both sides have the same solute concentration, they are isotonic.

If cells are placed in a hypertonic solution, movement of water will be out of the cell, causing the cell to shrivel. If cells are placed in a hypotonic solution, movement of water will be into the cell, causing the cell to swell or burst. Tonicity is useful only in reference to a particular cell or tissue.

Picture this: A man is about to put his contacts in when he realizes that he is out of contact solution. He finds a bottle of distilled water and decides to use the water for his contacts. His eyes get red and irritated and his contacts pop out. Why does this happen? Because the distilled water is hypotonic. His eyes are getting red because water is flowing into his cells and damaging those cells. Ideally, contact lens solution is isotonic—that is, a salt solution (NaCl) with the same osmolarity (discussed shortly) as is found in his extracellular tissues as well as inside his cells. The opposite situation would be placing a too-concentrated salt solution in the eyes. In this case, the salt solution is hypertonic and the eye's cells are damaged by too much water flowing out of them.

isotonic
describes a solution in which body cells can be bathed without net flow of water across the semipermeable cell membrane; also describes a solution with the same tonicity as another solution.

Isotonic solutions in the human body fall into the range of 280 to 310 milliosmoles per liter. Patient safety and comfort are best achieved by utilizing a solution that approximates this isotonic condition.

Osmolality and Osmolarity

Tonicity differs from osmolarity. Osmolarity is an absolute measure of the number of osmotically active solutes in a solution, whereas tonicity is a relative measure, based on the osmotic compatibility of a solution with a given cell type.

Let's begin with some useful definitions. A *mole* (abbreviated *mol*) is the amount of a substance that contains 6.022×10^{23} molecules (Avogadro's number). The mass in grams of one mole of a substance is the same as the number of atomic mass units in one molecule of that substance (that is, the molecular weight of the substance expressed as grams). The mole is the base unit in the SI system for the amount of a substance. An *osmole* is the amount of a solute that yields, in ideal solution, the number of particles (Avogadro's number) that would depress the freezing point of the solvent by 1.86 K.

Molality of a solution is the number of moles of a solute per *kilogram of solvent*

Molarity of a solution is the number of moles of solute per *litre of solution*

Osmolality of a solution is the number of osmoles of solute per *kilogram* of solvent

Osmolarity of a solution is the number of osmoles of solute per *litre* of solution

Osmolality depends on the number of particles (active ions or molecules) in a solution. It is commonly expressed as the number of milliosmoles of solute per kilogram of solvent (mOsm/kg).

Osmolarity is a measure of the osmotic pressure exerted by a solution across a perfect semipermeable membrane (one that allows free passage of water and completely prevents movement of solute) compared to pure water. It is commonly expressed as the number of milliosmoles of solute per liter of solution (mOsm/L).

osmolality
the concentration of solute in a solution per unit of solvent, commonly expressed as milliosmoles per kilogram

osmolarity
the concentration of solute in a solution per unit of solution; commonly expressed as milliosmoles per liter

ESTIMATING OSMOLARITY

It is important to know the osmolarity of a solution to avoid any potential problems with administering the IV solution. There are a number of ways to calculate this. The following is just one method for estimating the osmolarity of an IV solution.

1. For each component of the mixture, including sterile water, multiply the volume in milliliters of that component times the table value of milliosmoles present of the component.
2. Add the products obtained in step 1 for each of the components in order to determine the total number of milliosmoles in the mixture.
3. Add together each of the volumes in order to estimate the final total volume of the mixture.
4. Divide the total number of milliosmoles from step 2 by the total volume from step 3, then multiply by 1000 to estimate the osmolarity of the mixture in milliosmoles per liter.

EXAMPLE 4.1

Description	Volume	×	mOsm/mL	=	mOsm
Sterile water for injection	500 mL	×	0.00	=	0.00
Sodium bicarbonate 8.4%	50 mL	×	2.00	=	100.00
Potassium chloride	10 mL	×	4.00	=	40.00
Heparin 5,000 units	0.5 mL	×	0.46	=	0.23
Pyridoxine	1 mL	×	1.11	=	1.11
Thiamine	1 mL	×	0.62	=	0.62
Totals	553.50 mL				141.96
Osmolarity of admixture: (141.96/553.50) × 1000 = 256 mOsm/L					

SMALL-VOLUME PARENTERALS

Table 4.1 shows some values of mOsm/mL for common IV admixture components:

TABLE 4-1 Osmolarity of Small-Volume Parenterals

Description	mOsm/mL
Calcium chloride	2.04
Calcium gluconate	0.308
Cyanocobalamin (B-12)	0.45
Folic acid	0.20
Heparin	0.46
Lidocaine 2%	0.15
Magnesium sulfate	4.06
MVI 12 infusion (concentrate)	4.11
Potassium acetate	4.00
Potassium chloride	4.00
Potassium phosphate	7.4
Pyridoxine HCl (B-6)	1.11
Sodium acetate	4
Sodium bicarbonate 4.2%	1.00
Sodium bicarbonate 8.4%	2.00
Sodium chloride 14.6%	5
Sodium phosphate	12
Thiamine HCl (B-1)	0.62
Water for injection	0.00

LARGE-VOLUME PARENTERALS

Table 4.2 shows some values of mOsm/mL for common IV solutions:

TABLE 4-2 Osmolarity of Large-Volume Parenterals

Description	mOsm/mL
Sterile water	0.00
Dextrose 5%	0.25
Dextrose 10%	0.505
Dextrose 30%	1.51
Dextrose 50%	2.52
Dextrose 70%	3.53
Lactated Ringer's	0.28
Sodium chloride 0.45%	0.154
Sodium chloride 0.9%	0.31
Amino acid 8.5%	0.81
Amino acid 10%	0.998

CONCLUSION

Sterile products have special, unique properties that must be taken into consideration. Among the most crucial properties are pH, compatibility, stability, tonicity, osmolarity, and osmolality. Additional information on these properties is available in a number of pharmacy reference books, which should be available at any pharmacy preparing sterile products.

CHAPTER TERMS

acidic
describes a substance that increases the concentration of hydrogen ions (lowers the pH); an acidic substance is called an acid

alkaline
describes a substance that decreases the concentration of hydrogen ions (raises the pH); an alkaline substance is called a base

coring
transferring part of the rubber stopper of a vial or container into a solution bag because of improper needle stick

isotonic
describes a solution in which body cells can be bathed without net flow of water across the semipermeable cell membrane; also describes a solution with the same tonicity as another solution.

osmolality
the concentration of solute in a solution per unit of solvent; commonly expressed as milliosmoles per kilogram

osmolarity
the concentration of solute in a solution per unit of solution; commonly expressed as milliosmoles per liter

CHAPTER REVIEW QUESTIONS

MULTIPLE CHOICE

1. Water moves out of a cell, causing the cell to shrivel, when the cell is placed in a ________________ solution.
   a. isotonic
   b. hypotonic
   c. iso-osmotic
   d. hypertonic
   e. osmolality

2. Water moves into a cell, causing swelling, when the cell is placed in a ________________ solution.
   a. hypertonic
   b. isotonic
   c. tonicity
   d. hypotonic
   e. osmosis

3. If particulate matter enters and lodges in a vein, what could be the result? ________________.
   a. stroke
   b. inflammation
   c. sepsis
   d. both b and c
   e. both a and b

4. Human blood has a pH of ________________.
   a. 10.4
   b. 7.4
   c. 6.4
   d. 4.4
   e. 9.4

5. What are the three major types of incompatibilities? ________________.
   a. physical, chemical, therapeutic
   b. therapeutic, psychological, mechanical
   c. chemical, electrical, neurological
   d. physical, chemical, reactive
   e. therapeutic, medical, physical

6. A neutral solution is ________________.
   a. alkaline
   b. acidic
   c. chemically altered
   d. both a and b
   e. none of the above

7. What is the most likely reason that bar soap stings when it gets into the eyes? ________________.
   a. Water is added to the soap for lather.
   b. The pH balance is not equal between the eyes and the soap.
   c. The volume of the soap is greater than 5 g.
   d. The osmolarity is under 7.4.
   e. The pH of the soap is at 7.0.

8. In a hospital-type setting, sterile compounded products maintain an average shelf life of ________________.
   a. 10–12 hr
   b. 8–12 hr
   c. 4–6 hr
   d. 12–24 hr
   e. 24–48 hr

9. Sterile water has ________________ mOsm/mL.
   a. 15
   b. 0
   c. 5
   d. 10
   e. −0.5

10. If two solutions have the same solute concentration, they are known as ________________.
   a. isotonic
   b. hypertonic
   c. hypotonic
   d. iso-osmotic
   e. permeable

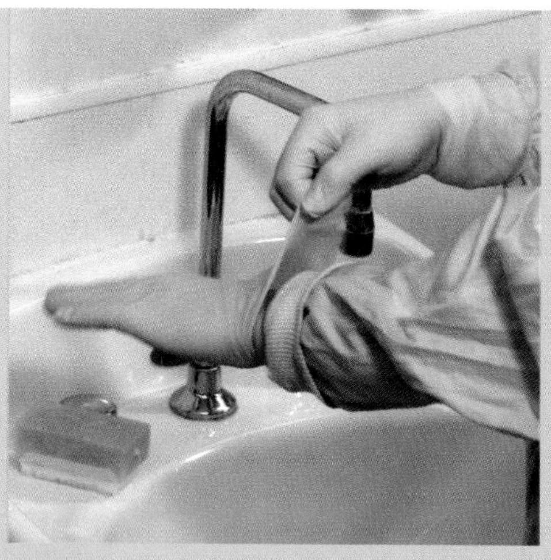

CHAPTER 5

Aseptic Technique

Learning Objectives

After completing this chapter, you should be able to:

- Explain how to design the clean room to limit contamination risk.
- Describe how to prepare vials, bags, and ampules before placing them in the airflow hood.
- Explain the theory of clean air space.
- Define and explain the importance of proper aseptic technique.
- Explain how to manipulate supplies such as needles, filters, and syringes.
- Manipulate specialty admix ingredients such as Factor VIII and Gammar globulin.
- Describe how to reconstitute a sterile product.

INTRODUCTION

Aseptic technique involves manipulating medications, fluids, and solutions and transferring them from one container to another, following stringent guidelines. Its primary goal is to keep cultures, sterile instruments, media, and people free of microbial contamination. Aseptic technique involves a lot of factors such as proper dress, hand washing, and manipulation. This chapter will touch on all the things a pharmacy technician should know before beginning to work in a clean room and environment.

Being physically able and technically correct to compound a sterile product is only a small part of the skill necessary to be competent in the IV room, however. The IV technician must have a wide variety of knowledge in such areas as terminology, IV room materials and supplies, proficiency with mathematical calculations, quality assurance, routes of administration, and drugs.

Preparation

As mentioned previously, appropriate dress must be worn at all times in the compounding area.

DRESSING

Dressing most commonly takes place in the anteroom. Articles worn may include specially designed lint-free paper gowns, paper hats (bouffant style), paper booties to cover shoes, jackets, face mask, paper arm guards, facial hair masks, and gloves (Figure 5-1). These types of dress are known as personal protective equipment (PPE).

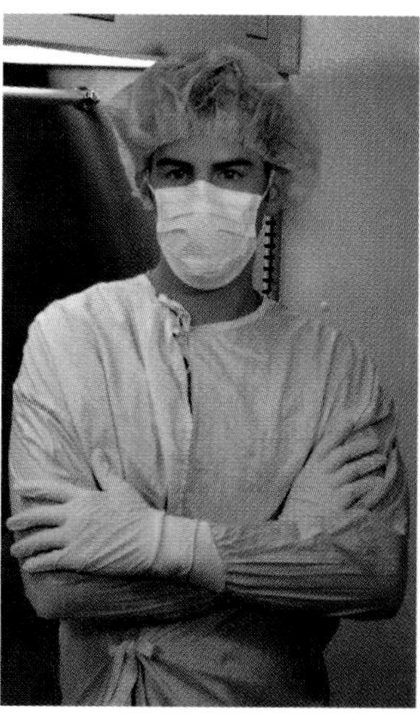

Figure 5-1 Proper dressing

HAND WASHING

Proper hand washing is important because all surfaces of our bodies have bacteria on them. These bacteria, called normal bacterial flora, typically do not affect healthy individuals. However, if the normal bacteria are accidentally given a little food (dextrose) and administered intravenously, they can and will cause an infection. If the patient is ill or **immunocompromised**, these normal bacteria will cause significant harm to the patient. In most institutions, gloves must also be worn. However, unless the gloves are sterile, the gloves must also be washed. Foaming alcohol may be used in between hand washings (for example, after answering a phone or using a computer); however, alcohol foam may not be used in place of regular hand washings.

immunocompromised a condition in which the immune system is not functioning normally

Here are some key points for hand washing (Figure 5-2):

- Wash your hands before entering the clean room, after eating, after performing any personal hygiene, or after doing anything that could cause contamination. You must do so before putting your hands in the hood.
- Use a germicidal, microbial soap, such as Hibiclens or chlorohexidene, to wash your hands thoroughly.
- Scrub with germicidal soap for at least 2 min, around and between all fingers and underneath fingernails. Scrub up to the elbow area of each arm, covering the entire area with soap, and rinse completely.
- Use lint-free paper towels to dry your hands after a hand washing. If the specially designed paper towels are not available, you may use gauze.

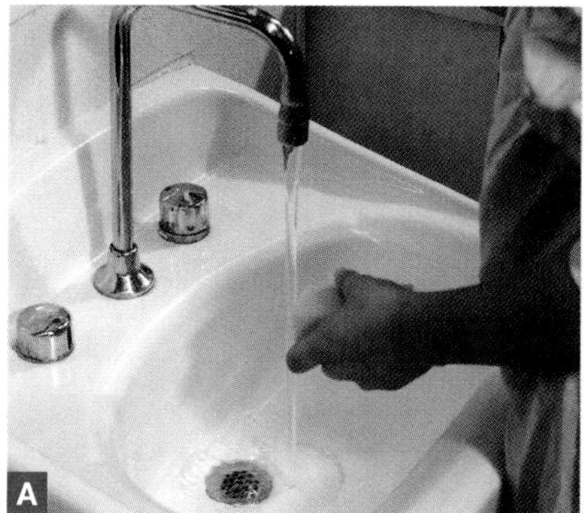

A

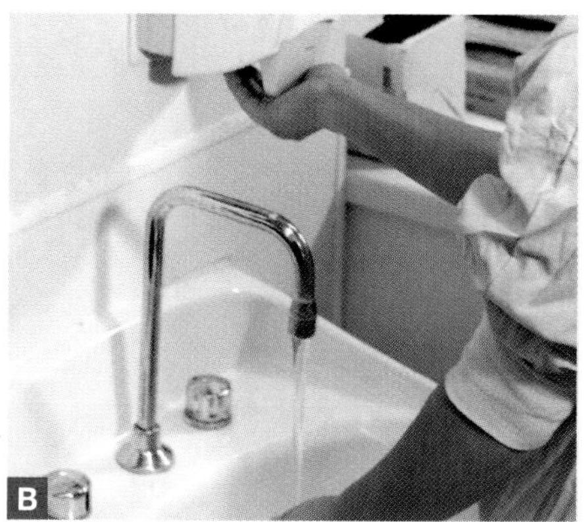

B

Figure 5-2 Proper hand washing

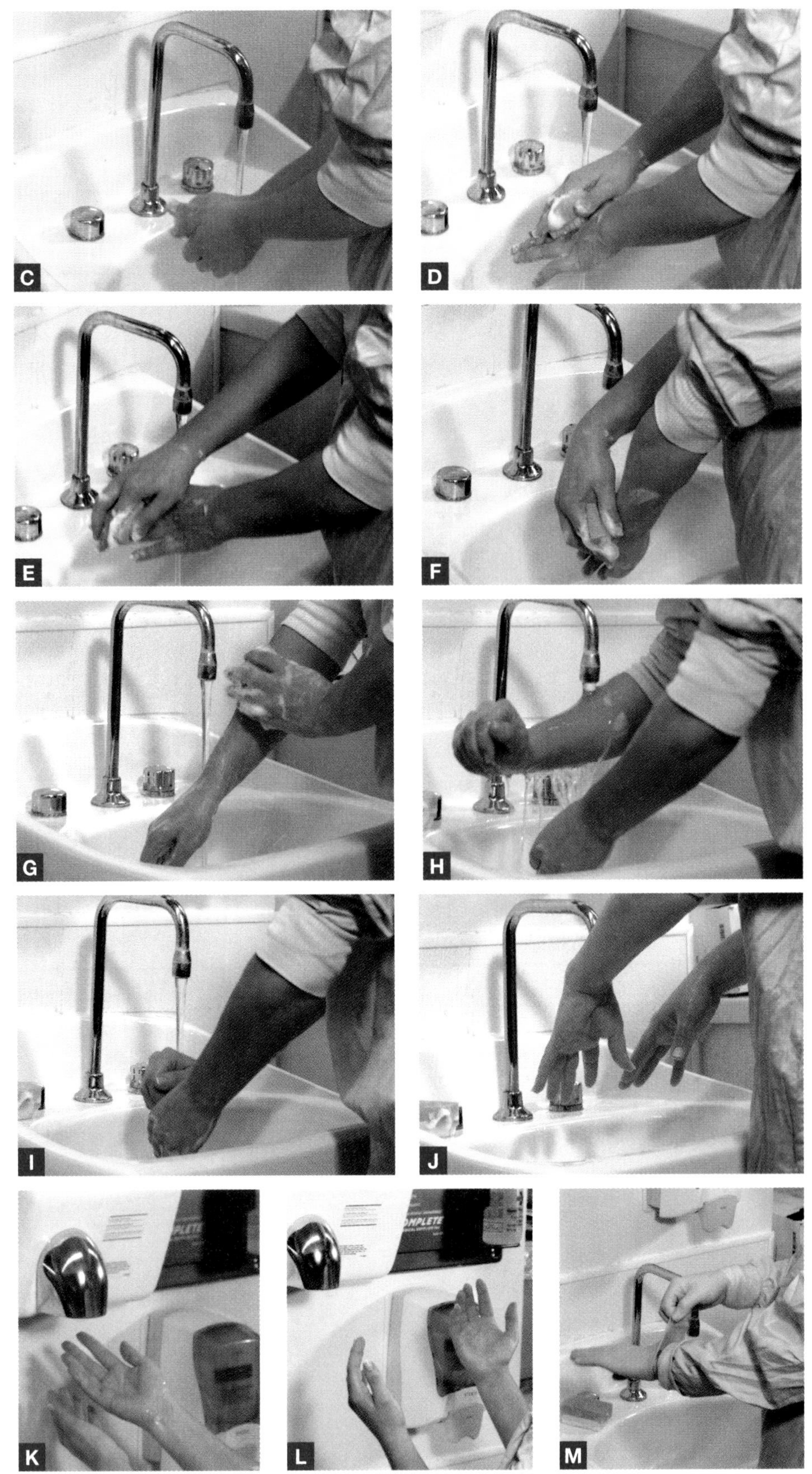

Figure 5-2 Proper hand washing (*continued*)

CLEAN ROOM

Access to the IV area should be limited to essential personnel only. No personnel should be allowed to approach the laminar airflow hood (LAH) unless properly gowned, adequately trained, and validated. Avoid horseplay or excessive movement near the hood, as this will disturb airflow.

Doors to the clean room must remain closed at all times. No food or drink is allowed in the IV room. Drinks must be kept in a sealed container outside the IV room. No gum chewing is allowed in the IV room. Avoid coughing, sneezing, singing, whistling, or excessive talking while under the hood because this may also contribute to adding contaminates to the air. Also, activities such as these can distract personnel, causing lost concentration and increasing the risk of medication errors (Figure 5-3).

USP 797 more specifically adds further restrictions, such as no jewelry, no fingernail polish or artificial nails, and no heavy makeup. The pharmacy technician should read and become very familiar with USP 797 and understand how it impacts the sterile product environment.

Externally clean and sanitize all supplies before bringing them into the clean room. Within this area you will uncarton, clean, and sanitize them and then transfer them to a clean cart restricted to the controlled area.

A further transfer barrier step should occur as supply items are introduced into the LAH. Whenever possible, remove external wrappings (such as IV outerbags and syringe pouches) at the edge of the LAH. Limit supply items introduced into the LAH to those required for the planned procedure, and arrange them so as not to obstruct the HEPA airflow pattern and to provide for efficient processing.

Figure 5-3 Clean room

CLEAN AIR SPACE

You must perform all compounding at least 6 in. inside the edges of the LAH; this area is known as the clean air space. As the sterile air hits the sides of the LAH, the air is considered contaminated and no longer clean. As the air moves toward the outer edge of the hood, the room air begins to mix with the clean air, reducing sterility.

Just as the technician has appropriately prepared, the LAH must also be prepared. The blower should remain on at all times. If it has been turned off, it must remain on at least 30 min prior to use. The LAH must be cleaned with 70% isopropyl alcohol or another sanitizing agent using a lint-free wipe or gauze.

Proper Aseptic Technique

Following is the how-to of aseptic technique and some special considerations for dealing with different products. Read this section carefully, as it is very important for you to become proficient in this task. Refer to this section as often as necessary throughout your pharmacy career. With time and experience, you should become proficient and knowledgeable as you work with many types of fluids, medications, and equipment.

MANIPULATION

To maintain sterility, you must avoid touching several areas during sterile product manipulations and preparation. Avoid direct contact with any previously swabbed area (vial top, bag port, neck of an ampule), uncapped needles, the hub of the needle, the syringe tip, the syringe plunger, the open tip of a filter or dispensing pin, and the uncapped tip of any tubing.

Basically, any area that may come in contact with the sterile solution should not come in contact with any nonsterile area, including hands, fingers, or any parts that can come in contact with hands and fingers. As a general rule, if the manufacturer has made a cover for a part on a syringe or tubing, that part should remain untouched and sterile. All syringes must have a capped needle or a syringe cap on before you lay them on the hood's surface. Never place uncapped needles or uncovered syringes in the hood.

When withdrawing solution using a dispensing pin, place the dispensing pin cap on a clean alcohol swab. Immediately recap the solution after use and discard the swab.

Swabbing with Alcohol

To guarantee sterility of an area that will be punctured/penetrated by a needle, tubing, and so on, you must swab it with 70% isopropyl alcohol. Areas that must be swabbed include the following:

- vial tops
- ampule necks
- tops of bottles
- ports of any IV or IVPB bags

To properly use an alcohol pad, place the alcohol pad on the area to be swabbed, allowing it to remain for several seconds or until the surface becomes saturated with alcohol. Then make one gentle stroke across the area to be cleaned, moving the swab toward either the side or the front of the hood (not toward the HEPA filter). Use a clean, saturated, unused portion of the swab with each pass. Be certain to allow the alcohol to dry fully before use. Swabbing is effective in two important ways—removing any physical contaminants such as dust and acting as a disinfectant because the evaporation of alcohol, called desiccation, creates sterility.

Using Syringes

Syringes are available in numerous sizes with volumes ranging from 0.5 mL to 60 mL. To maximize accuracy, use the smallest syringe size that can hold the desired amount of solution. According to ASHP guidelines, the total volume being measured must be at least 20 percent of the total size of the syringe. This is known as the 20 percent rule. To maintain sterility, two parts of the syringe cannot be touched—the tip and the plunger.

Syringes are single-dose items that you must dispose of in the sharps container after use. You must open the syringe package within the clean air space in the LAH in order to maintain sterility. Do not place the syringe's outer packaging on the working surface of the LAH because it will contaminate the hood's surface. Place the outer covering directly into the garbage after removing the syringe.

Syringes are packaged with either a needle and cap or a protective cover over the tip. Do not remove the protective tip cover until a new needle is ready to be attached on the tip of the syringe. If the syringe does not come with either a protective cap or a capped needle, you must attach a new needle on the syringe immediately, before laying the syringe on the hood's surface.

Many syringes have locking mechanisms, such as a leur-lock at the tip that secures the needle by allowing it to be screwed down onto a threaded ring. When you attach a needle to a leur-lock type syringe, you must turn the needle slightly to ensure a tight fit. In other cases, the needle is held on only by friction; these are known as slip tips.

Using Needles

Many needles are available in different sizes and lengths. The width of a needle is measured in gauges. The larger the gauge of a needle, the smaller the bore (width). For example, a 27-gauge needle has a smaller bore than a 13-gauge needle. Handle a needle only by the protective cover. Avoid touching the hub of a needle.

Using Vials

Date all vials before you bring them into the hood. Single-dose vials contain no preservatives and should be discarded at the end of the shift. There are several situations in which you must use a preservative-free vial, such as pediatric dilutions, epidurals, and intrathecals. Medications with preservatives can seriously harm patients if administered in these situations.

Multiple-dose vials contain preservatives that allow their contents to be used after the vial has been punctured. These vials each have specific instructions outlined in the package inserts that describe how the vial should be kept (for example, refrigerated) and for how long the vial remains stable. Consult a pharmacist if there are questions regarding the vial's stability. But remember, "When in doubt, toss it out."

When a vial is pierced by a needle, *cores* or fragments of the rubber stopper can form. To prevent this problem, insert the needle into the rubber stopper with the bevel tip up, then apply a slight lateral pressure (away from the bevel) and downward pressure to insert the needle. Make sure to maintain aseptic technique and avoid shadowing at all times.

Vials are closed-system containers because air cannot flow freely into or out of the vial. Therefore, adding air or fluid to a closed system will cause the vial to become pressurized, also known as *positive pressure*. Positive pressure can cause some spraying of the fluid from the vial or can cause the vial to become leaky. On the other hand, removing air or fluid from the vial can create a vacuum in the vial. If too much of a vacuum is created, it is nearly impossible to remove the contents of the vial aseptically. Therefore, the volume of the fluid to be removed from a vial should be replaced with a slightly smaller volume of air to minimize the vacuum. It is better to have a slight vacuum in a vial because it results in a cleaner withdrawal. Do not add air to gas-producing drugs such as ceftazidime or any chemotherapy drugs.

If the drug within the vial is in a powdered form, it must first be **reconstituted**. Reconstitution is the adding of a diluent to a vial to create a liquid

reconstitute
to add a diluent to a vial to create a liquid

form of the drug. The desired volume of the diluting solution or diluent, usually SWFI (sterile water for injection), is injected into the vial. As the diluent is added, an equal volume of air must be removed to prevent positive pressure from building up within the vial. This is accomplished by allowing an equal amount of air to flow back into the syringe that was used to reconstitute the vial or by using a vented needle. A vented needle allows free flow of air out of the vial during reconstitution, resulting in the release of the built-up positive pressure.

Although most drugs dissolve rapidly when swirled, the IV tech must make sure that a drug is completely dissolved before proceeding. Visually inspect all reconstituted drugs to ensure that the powder is completely dissolved and that there are no cores or other particulate matter in the solution. Carefully inspect the container fully, including as close to the needle entrance as possible and behind any ridges. If you observe or suspect any particulate matter, filter the solution before adding it to the final parenteral product.

PERFORMING A STRAIGHT DRAW

This type of manipulation is the simplest and most common. It can be used in almost all manipulations in one form or another.

Procedure

You must perform a straight draw procedure in the clean air space using proper aseptic technique (Figure 5-4):

1. Gather all materials needed for the manipulation.
2. Swab the rubber top with alcohol. Allow the alcohol to dry.
3. Make sure the needle is firmly attached to the syringe.
4. Pull the plunger back on the syringe to slightly less than the amount needed to be drawn up.

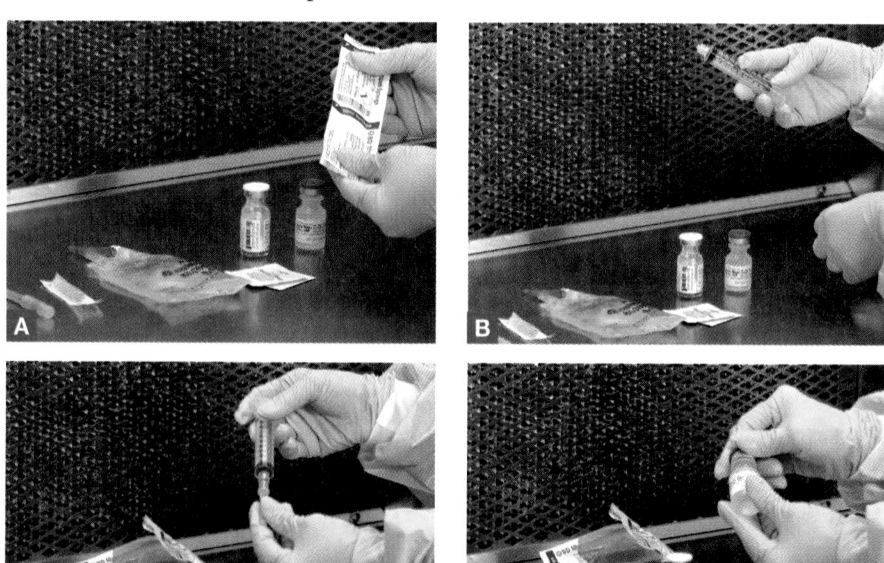

Figure 5-4 Straight draw

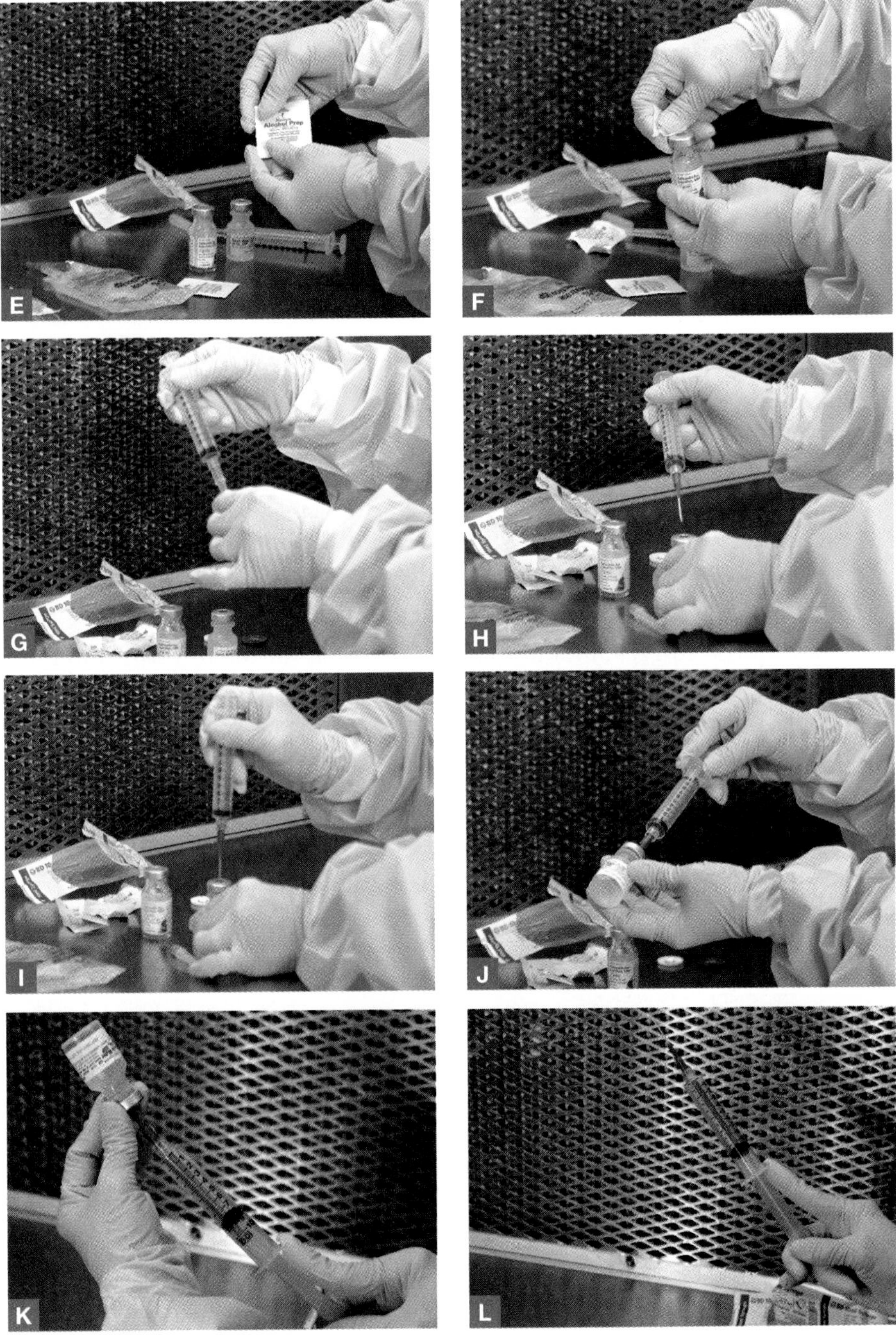

Figure 5-4 Straight draw *(continued)*

5. Remove the needle cap. Find the center of the stopper and position the needle with the bevel end up.
6. Slightly bend the needle and insert the needle through the stopper.
7. Gently push the air from the syringe into the vial.
8. Pull back on the stopper until the desired amount is withdrawn.
9. Remove any air bubbles.
10. Withdraw the needle and carefully recap.

RECONSTITUTING A POWDERED VIAL

Materials

- powdered vial
- diluent vial (usually sterile water for injection)
- alcohol swabs
- appropriate size syringes
- vented needle
- two regular needles
- IV bag

Procedure

You must perform the reconstituting a powdered vial procedure in the clean air space using proper aseptic technique (Figure 5-5).

1. Gather all materials needed for the manipulation.
2. Swab all rubber tops with alcohol. Allow the alcohol to dry.
3. Make sure the needle is firmly attached to the syringe.
4. Draw up the correct amount of diluent needed for the reconstitution.
5. Pull back on the plunger to clear the neck of the syringe. Remove the needle and replace with a vented needle.
6. Carefully add diluent to the powdered vial.
7. Gently shake or swirl to dissolve. The powder must dissolve completely.
8. Either get a new syringe or change the vented needle back to a regular needle and carefully remove the desired amount from the vial.
9. Remove any air bubbles.
10. Insert the needle into the additive port of the IV bag and slowly inject.

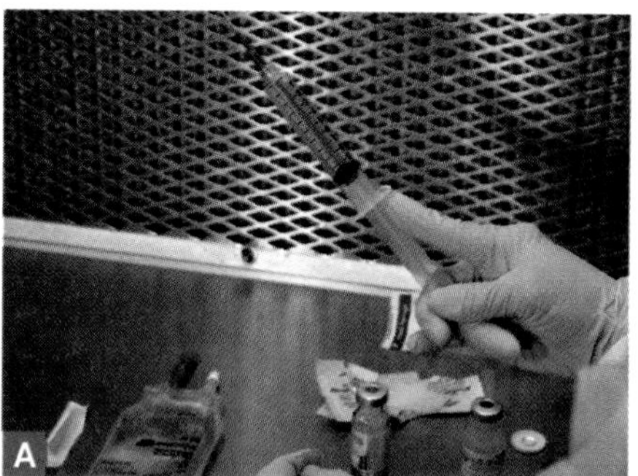

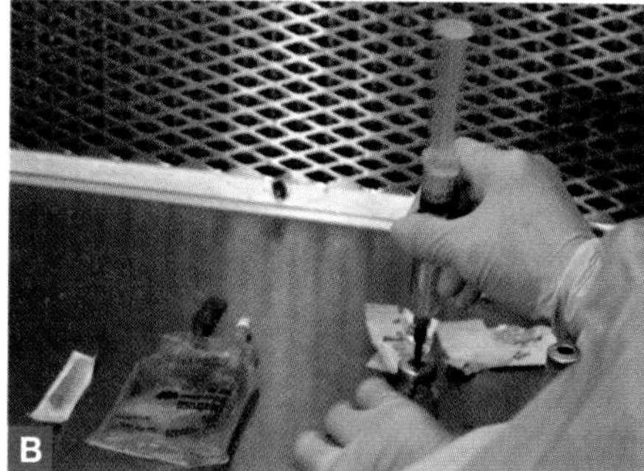

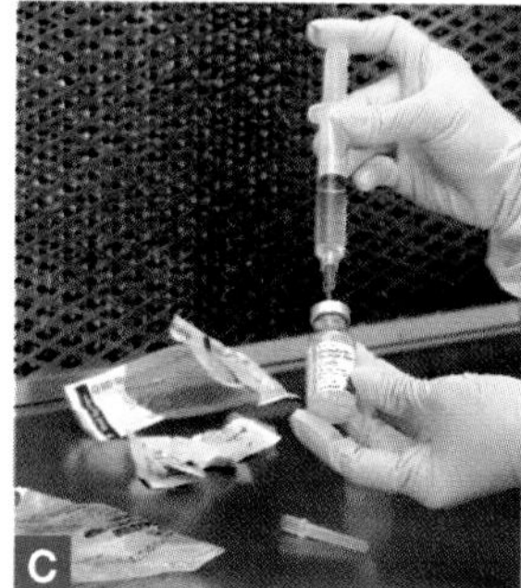

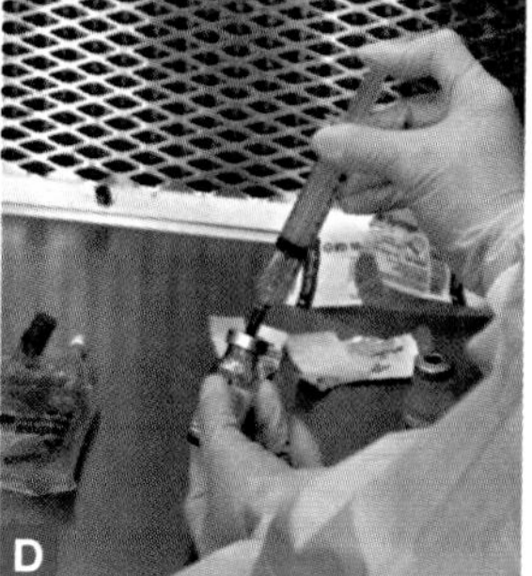

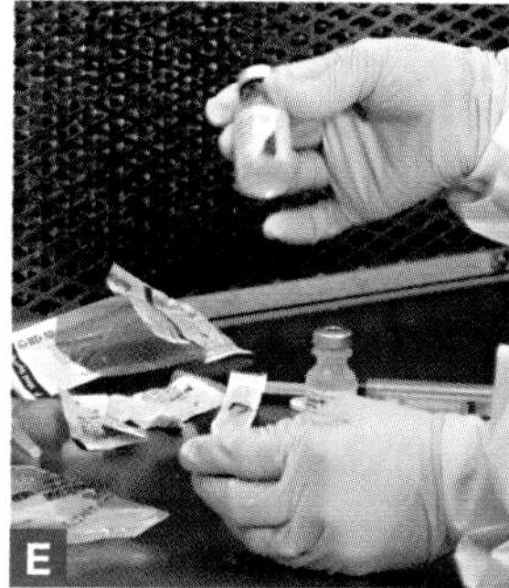

Figure 5-5
Reconstitution of a vial

MORE ON MANIPULATION

Removing Air Bubbles

Often air bubbles will be present in the syringe after you have drawn up the medication (Figure 5-6). To remove air bubbles, draw back on the plunger to allow more air in the syringe. Then carefully rotate the large air bubble around the syringe. Hopefully the larger air bubble will pick up most of the smaller air bubbles. If air bubbles are left, carefully tap the syringe to dislodge the smaller air bubbles. Hold the syringe upright and pull the plunger back another 0.2 mL (to clear the hub). Then carefully push the plunger up to remove the air. Make sure that the desired amount is left in the syringe. This manipulation can be performed only in a closed system, which means with the cap on the needle.

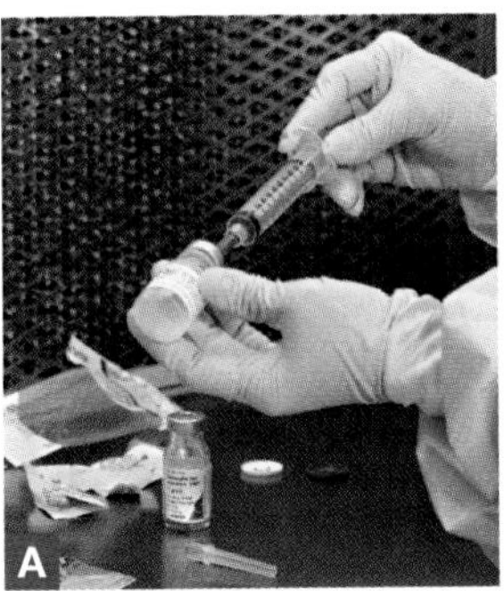

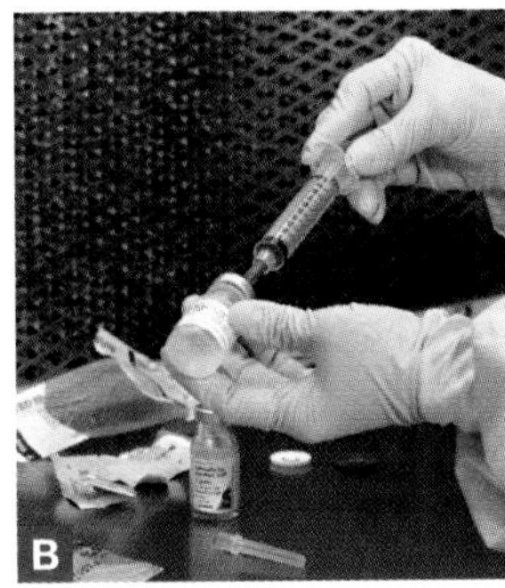

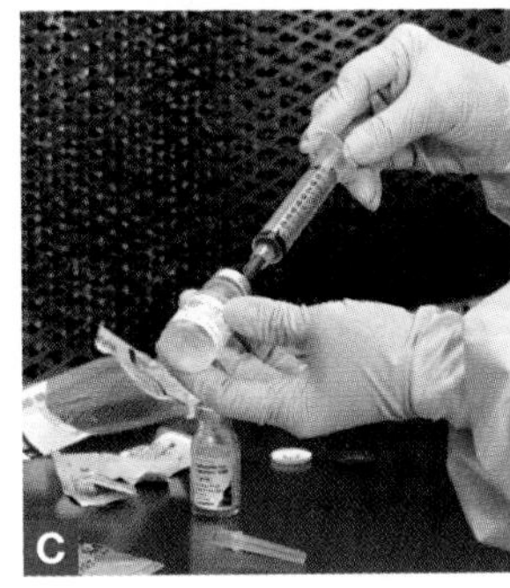

Figure 5-6 Removing air bubble

Using Transfer Needles

Transfer needles are double-ended, which means they have needles on both ends. Transfer needles are useful when the entire contents of a vial are going to be transferred into an IVPB. For example, if you have a vial of Rocephin 1 g IVPB, the entire gram of Rocephin will be reconstituted and added to an IVPB.

To use a tranfer needle (Figure 5-7), swab the appropriate areas and place the longer of the two ends in the additive port of the IVPB. Place the shorter end in the desired vial. The transfer needle connects the bag and the vial, allowing the fluid to flow between them. Gently squeeze the IV bag and the IV fluid will slowly fill the vial. Shake the vial gently until all of the powder is dissolved. When all the powder is dissolved, hold the IV bag so that all of the air floats to the top, then gently squeeze the bag. This process will cause the air to move into the vial, thus creating pressure in the vial. The pressure will force the fluid down into the bag. Since the addition of Add-A-Vials and Advantage vials, transfer needles are not being used as often as they once were.

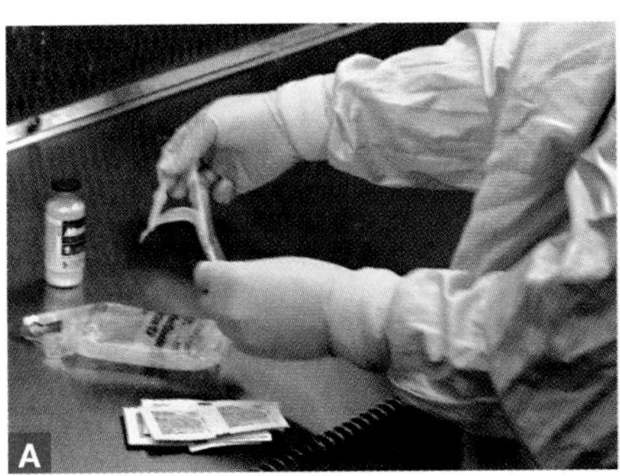

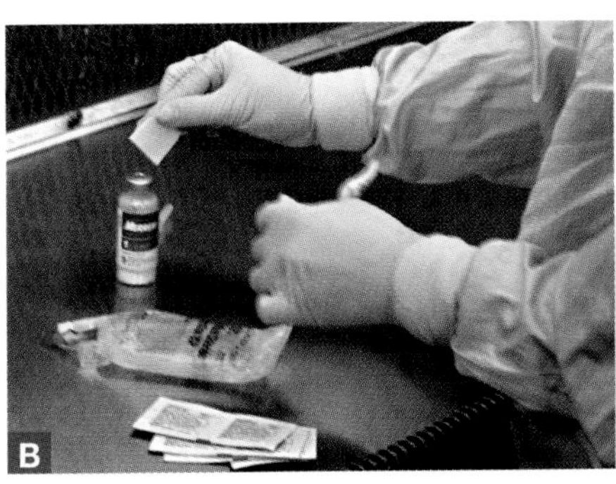

Figure 5-7 Using a transfer needle

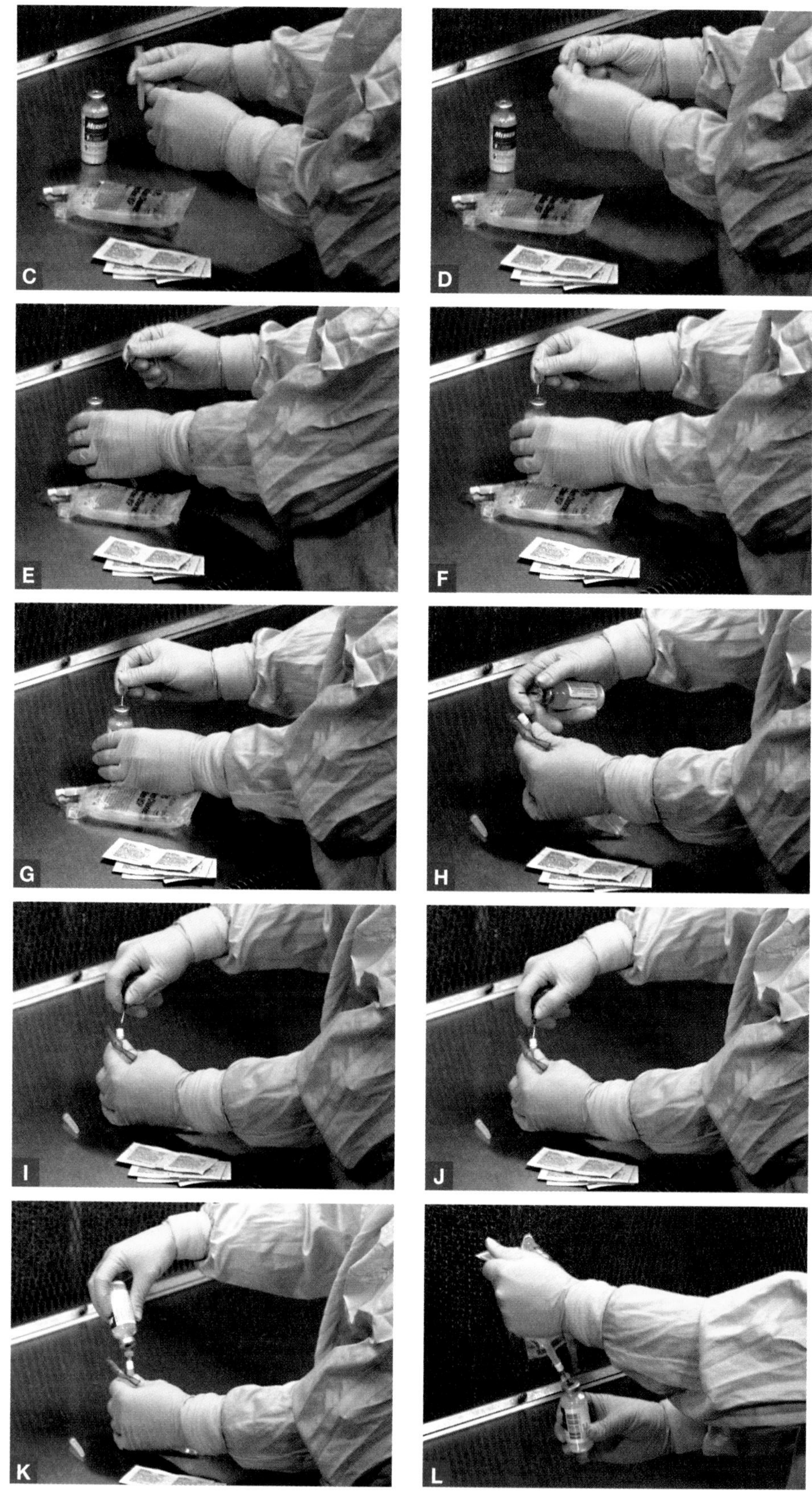

Figure 5-7 Using a transfer needle (*continued*)

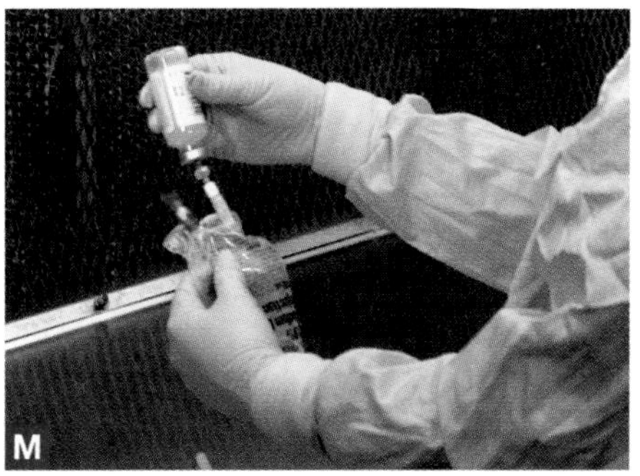

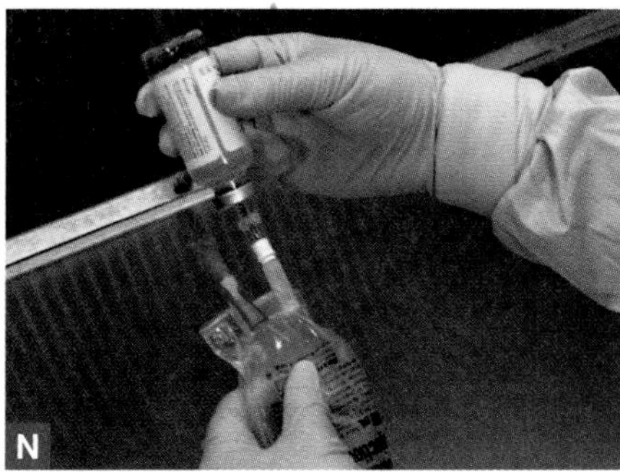

Figure 5-7 Using a transfer needle *(continued)*

Using Ampules

Unlike vials, ampules are composed entirely of glass. After an ampule is opened, it becomes an open system and a single-use container. Because the ampule is an open system (air can pass freely into and out of the ampule), the volume of the fluid removed does not have to be replaced with air. Before an ampule is opened, all the fluid must be moved from the head and neck (top part) to the body (lower part). This can be accomplished by one of the following methods: swirling the ampule in an upright motion, tapping the head of the ampule with a finger, or inverting the ampule and then quickly swinging it to an upright position. Sometimes one of these methods may be used and sometimes all three of these methods may be used.

To open an ampule properly, swab the neck of the ampule with alcohol and allow the alcohol to dry. Place a clean alcohol swab on the neck of the ampule. This swab can help prevent accidental cuts to the finger as well as minimize the spraying of glass particles and aerosolized drug. Place the head of the ampule between the thumb and the index finger on one hand, and hold the body of the ampule by the thumb and index finger of the other hand. Usually, right-handed people hold the top of the ampule with their right hand. However, do what is comfortable. If the ampule has a dot on it, face the dot away from the direction in which the ampule is being broken. The dot indicates a weak area on the neck of the ampule. Exert pressure on both thumbs, pushing the ampule away from yourself in a quick snapping motion. This pressure should cause the neck of the ampule to break (Figure 5-8).

Open ampules only to the side of the hood and never toward the HEPA filter (back of the hood). If an ampule is broken toward the back of the hood, small glass particles can damage the HEPA filter. Extreme pressure may crush the ampule. If the ampule does not break easily, rotate the ampule so that the pressure on the neck of the ampule is at a different angle.

To withdraw fluid from the ampule, tilt the ampule downward slightly so that you can place the bevel of a needle in the inside bottom corner of the ampule. Once the fluid covers the bevel of the needle, pull back on the syringe's plunger to withdraw the solution. Since glass particles may have

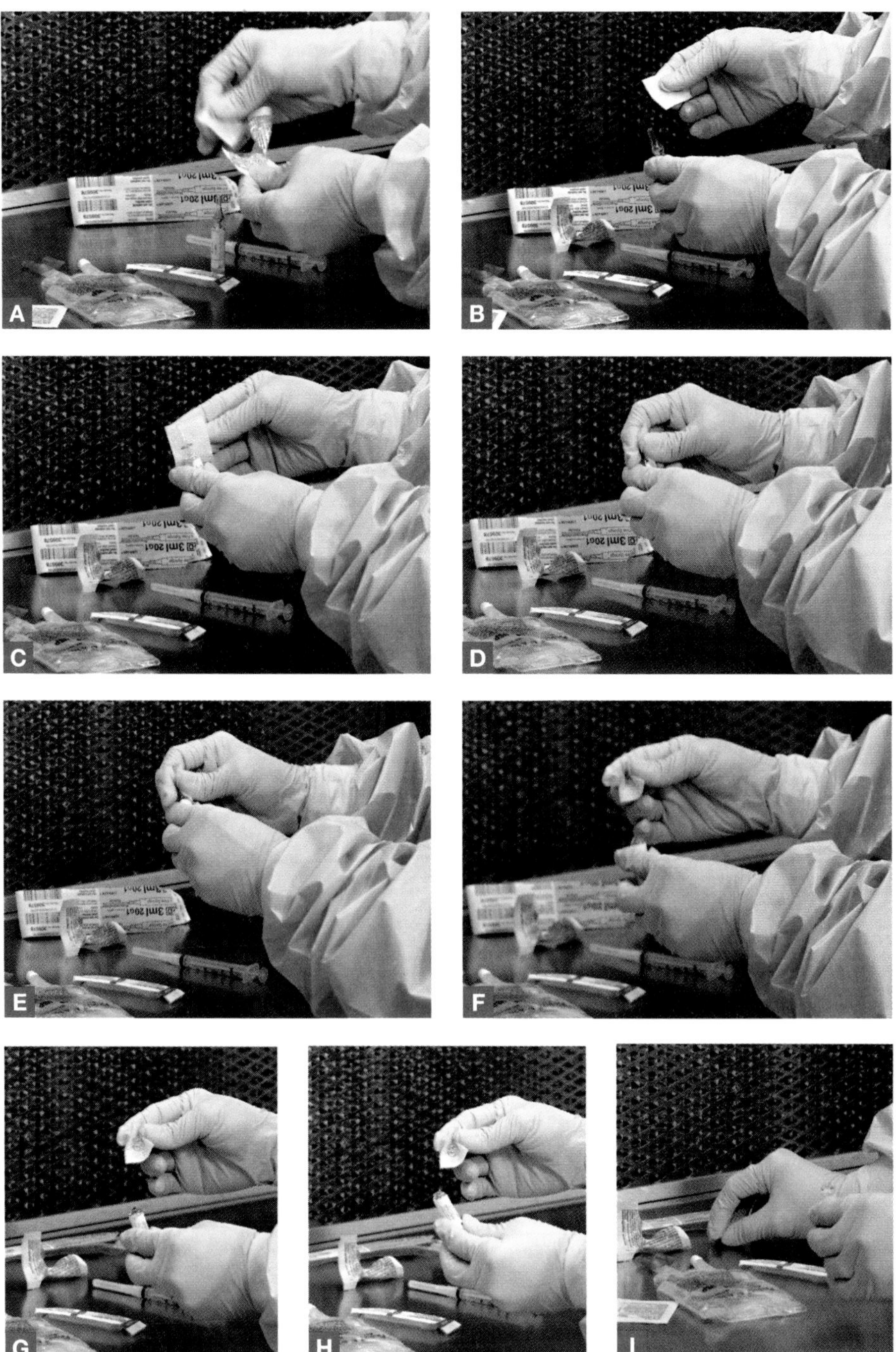

Figure 5-8 Opening an ampule

entered the solution as you broke the ampule, you must filter the solution before adding it to a bag. There are several ways to do this (Figure 5-9):

- Draw the medication into a syringe through a filter needle, then change to a regular needle to add the bag.
- Draw the medication into a syringe through a regular needle, then change to a filter needle to add to the bag.

- Draw the medication up using a filter straw (useful for tall ampules), then change to a regular needle to add to the bag.
- Draw the medication up into a syringe using a regular needle, then push it through an IVEX filter.

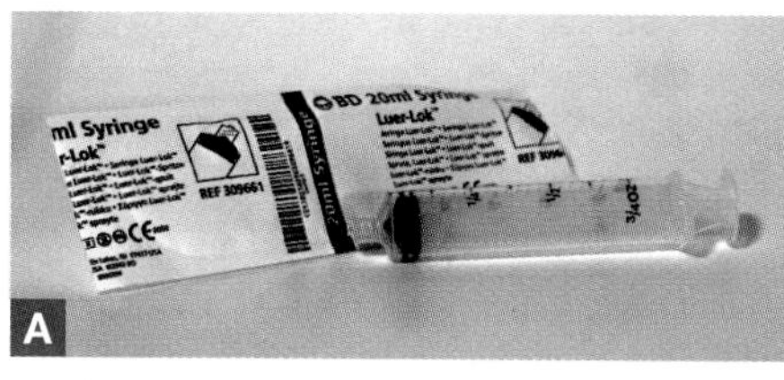

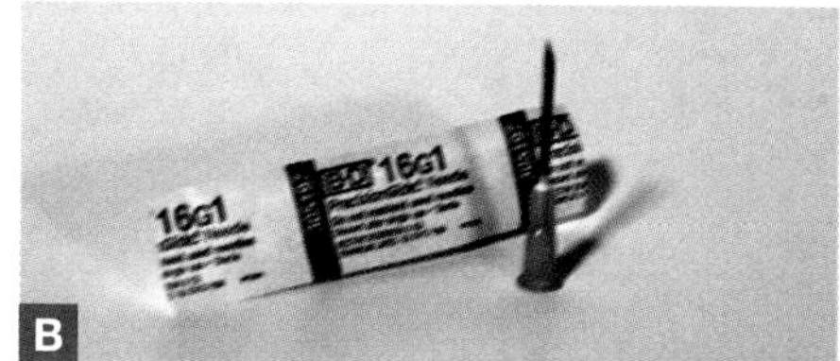

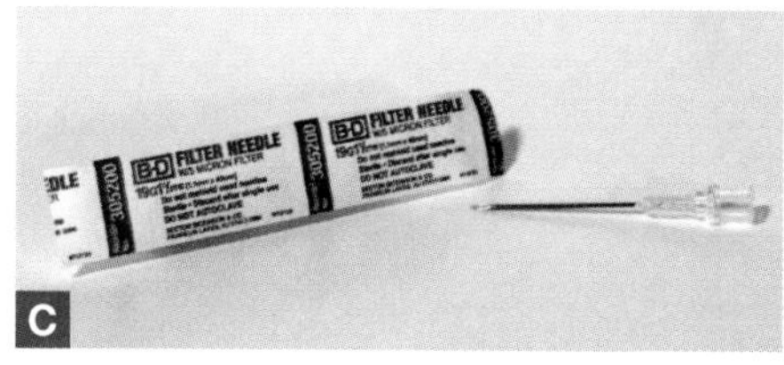

Figure 5-9 Filtration methods

REMOVING FLUID FROM AN AMPULE

Materials

alcohol swabs
ampule(s)
filter needle
regular needle
appropriate size syringe
IV bag or syringe cap

Procedure

You must perform this procedure in the clean air space using proper aseptic technique (Figure 5-10):

1. Gather all materials needed for the manipulation.
2. Remove any fluid from the neck of the ampule.
3. Swab the neck with alcohol.
4. Hold the ampule at a 20-degree angle toward the side of the hood.
5. Using your thumbs, apply pressure toward the neck of the ampule.
6. Change the needle on the syringe to a filter needle. Withdraw the fluid using a filter needle.
7. Remove any air bubbles.
8. Change the needle to a regular needle before injecting into a bag.
9. Remove any air bubbles.
10. Insert the needle into the additive port of the IV bag and slowly inject.

WORKPLACE WISDOM

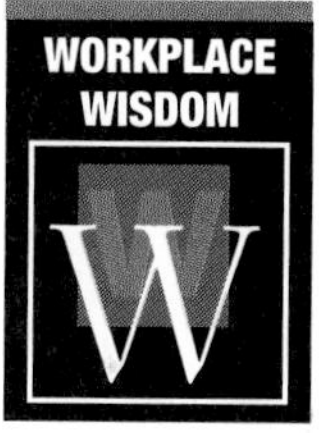

In all cases, do not use the same needle used to withdraw the fluid from the ampule to inject it into an IV bag. A filter needle can be used only once. Using it twice, to withdraw and to inject, will nullify the filtering effort.

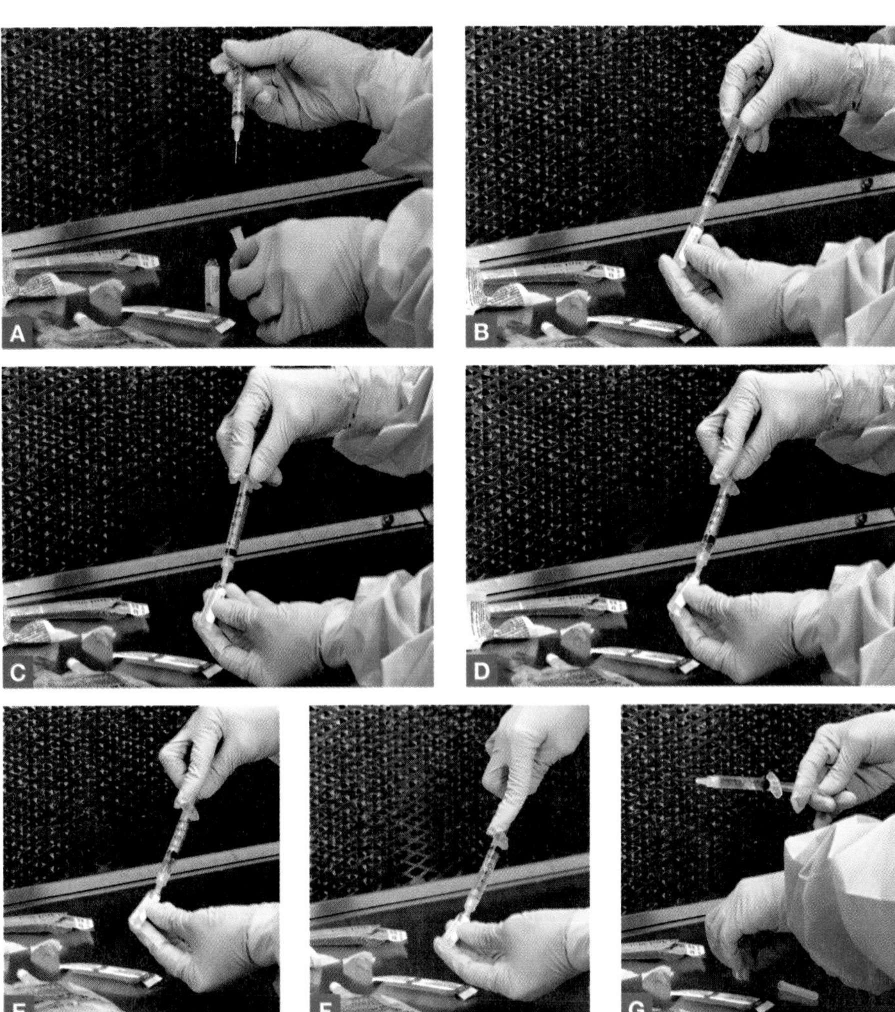

Figure 5-10 Withdrawing fluid from an ampule

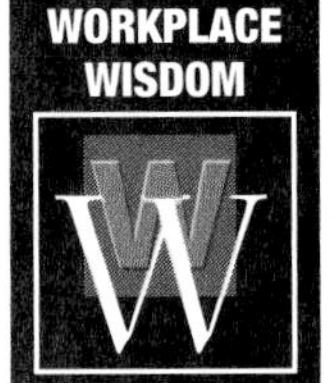

Never pick up a needle cap in one hand and use it to recap an exposed needle in another hand during the mixing process. Instead, leave the cap in the package inside the hood while mixing, then when ready, slip the needle into the cap and then use the other hand to secure the cap. This prevents unwanted and dangerous needle sticks.

PREPARING A STERILE DOSAGE FORM

Procedure

Sterile dosage forms may be prepared in various final containers, including flexible plastic bags, glass bottles, glass vials, semirigid plastic containers, and syringes. Before compounding, assemble all materials. Place only necessary materials within the LAH (Figure 5-11).

Next, clean all injection surfaces with a 70% alcohol swab. After the alcohol has dried, withdraw drug fluids aseptically from the containers in the amounts needed, using the appropriate size syringe. Once all the drug fluids are drawn up, place the syringes with the needles capped on the surface of the hood next to the medication vial. Next to the syringe, place the appropriate base solution. Check the label again to make sure the correct additives and amounts are drawn up and the correct base is present. If everything is correct, circle the amount being added. Depending on the institutional policy, a pharmacist may be required to check the additives before they are injected into the base. Needles must be carefully inserted into the port of a bag so that the needle does not puncture the bag. If the preparation that is being compounded is a pediatric preparation, a narcotic, a chemotherapy preparation, or a TPN, a pharmacist should check the additives before they are added to the base.

Since large amounts of water and potassium chloride are used during the day, these solutions, attached to transfer tubing, are often hanging in the hood. This enables the technician to draw up large volumes of these solutions very easily. They are easily accessible for STAT preparations. Large glass bottles (empty evacuated containers, or EECs) contain a very strong vacuum; therefore, you should never add KCl (potassium chloride) or water to them using a transfer set. The vacuum will continue to draw fluid into the bottle and has the potential to create very dangerous errors in dosing. Therefore, you must draw up SWFI and KCl using individual syringes. Position the injection port of a bag, covered by a protective tip, toward the HEPA filter when preparing an IV admixture, to maintain sterility. If you are using a glass bottle, remove the aluminum cap and place the bottle 6 in. away from the HEPA filter.

Nothing must come between the HEPA filter and the port to which additives are added (this includes vials, syringes, and hands). Disinfect all injection surfaces by swabbing the surface with 70% alcohol and allowing the alcohol to dry. Insert the needle into the rubber stopper or latex diaphragm. Insert needles carefully using a noncoring technique, as described earlier. After you inject the additive, reswab the port with alcohol. Then cover the top of the glass bottle with an IVA seal before removing it from the hood. Once the sterile product is compounded, properly label it and inspect it for cores and particulate matter. If a check has not already been made, place the final solution on the counter with all its contributors and appropriate syringes.

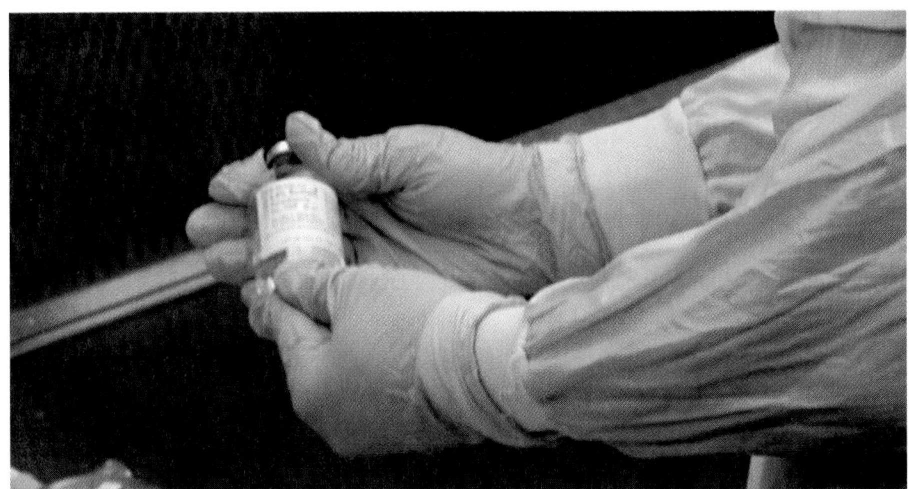

Figure 5-11 Preparing a sterile product

Special Preparations

Special preparations include blood products, product descriptions, and handling information.

FACTOR VIII, FACTOR IX, AND OTHER BLOOD PRODUCTS

Several blood products are used in the institutional pharmacy. Some of the most familiar blood products that are used in pharmacies have been treated to reduce the risk of transmitting viral infections, such as HIV or hepatitis. However, the risk of viral contamination from these products cannot be entirely eliminated. For this reason, use special care and handling procedures while working with blood products. It is advisable to read the package insert for any blood products before working with them because different manufacturers may have different guidelines for handling, reconstituting and stability.

PRODUCT DESCRIPTION AND HANDLING INFORMATION

Albumin (Albuminar, Albutein)

Albumin is a sterile solution for a single-dose administration, containing 25% human albumin. Albumin is used to treat hypovolemic shock, in conjunction with exchange transfusion, in the treatment of neonatal hyperbilirubinemia, and for other conditions.

Albumin can be a floor stock item in critical-care areas. In most cases, albumin will be sent to the floor in the original package. Make sure to send the enclosed plastic bag to the floor along with the vial; it is used to administer the albumin to the patient. Do not use albumin solutions if they appear turbid or if there is sediment in the bottle. Begin administration within 4 hr after the bottle is punctured. Dispose of empty albumin vials in an approved sharps container.

Plasma Protein Fraction (PPF)

PPF is a sterile solution for single-dose intravenous administration containing 5% plasma proteins. PPF is used to prevent and treat hypovolemic shock and in cases of severe hypoproteinuria, as in adjunct hemodialysis. PPF is floor stocked in the intensive care nursery. In most cases, PPF will be sent to the floor in the original vial. Do not use solutions of PPF if they appear turbid or if there is sediment in the bottle. Begin administration within 4 hr after the container has been entered. Dispose of empty PPF vials in an approved sharps container.

Immunoglobulin (Gammar, IgG)

Immune globulin intravenous is a sterile, lyophilized, single-dose preparation of immune globulin. Gammar is indicated for patients with primary defective or suppressed immune systems, who are at increased risk of infection. Wear chemo gloves when preparing this product. Do not mix immune globulin products of differing formulations. In other words, do not mix two different brands of IgG.

IgG must be reconstituted before being administered. Most IgG preparations include a double-ended, vented spike adapter with a plastic piercing pin. It is very important to use the transfer pins correctly. Failure to follow the reconstitution instructions could lead to contamination of the product and/or loss of vacuum, which would make IgG impossible to reconstitute. Read the package insert for step-by-step reconstitution instructions. Do not shake the product vial, as excessive foaming and protein bruising will occur. Gently swirl the vial once the diluent has been added. Use within 24 hr of reconstitution, or as recommended by the package insert. Visually inspect the solution for any particulate matter and discoloration prior to administration. Dispose of empty IgG containers, tubings, and so on in an approved sharps container. Pharmacy personnel should deliver IgG preparations to the floor, or the nurse should pick them up. Do not tube IgG preparations. Check with the nurse before making any scheduled doses, as Gammar has a short stability time and is very expensive.

Factor VIII (Alphanate)

Factor VIII is a sterile, lyophilized, single-dose concentrate of antihemophilic factor (AHF). Factor VIII is used to prevent and control bleeding in patients with Factor VIII deficiency due to hemophilia-A or acquired Factor VIII deficiency. Wear chemo gloves when preparing this product. Do not mix Factor VIII products from differing formulations; in other words, do not mix different brands of Factor VIII in the same container.

Factor VIII is ordered in units. Lyophilized Factor VIII concentrate is available in many different sizes. The number of units in the vial varies with each lot number. When preparing Factor VIII, try to come as close as possible to the number of units that the physician orders. If it is impossible to get the exact number of units ordered, always go over; never go under the amount of units that the physician orders. For example, if the physician orders 1000 units and the pharmacy has only two 510-unit vials and two 480-unit vials, use the two 510 vials for a total of 1020 units rather than having 990 units.

Always draw up the complete vial; never use a partial vial in an attempt to get an exact dose. Label the dose with the exact amount contained in the syringe. Factor VIII is usually stored in the refrigerator (some brands are stored in the freezer); whenever possible, remove the Factor VIII from the refrigerator approximately 30 min before reconstitution. This allows the concentrate and the diluent to warm to room temperature and helps the concentrate dissolve more easily. Reconstitute the concentrate according to the package insert instructions. Do not shake the reconstituted product, as excessive foaming will result. Gently swirl the contents once the diluent has been added. Withdraw the reconstituted product into a syringe through the vented filter spike provided in the package. Whenever possible, do not fill the syringe to more than two-thirds of its maximum capacity.

Before capping with a red leur-lock syringe cap, draw approximately 10 cc of air into the syringe. This will reduce bubbling and foaming and, more important, will reduce the risk of exposure to nursing staff if the AHF leaks into the cap or the transport bag. Administer Factor VIII within 8 hr or as directed in the package insert. Discard all empty AHF vials and associated tubing, equipment, and so on into an approved sharps container. Factor VIII should be delivered by pharmacy personnel or picked up by a nurse. Do not tube AHF.

Check with the nurse before making any scheduled doses of Factor VIII since this product has a short stability, is extremely expensive, and is very unlikely to be able to be used on another patient. Notify your supervisor immediately upon accidental exposure to AHF products.

Factor IX (Konyne)

Factor IX is a sterile, lyophilized, single-dose concentrate of AHF intended for IV administration to treat Factor IX deficiency. The reconstitution, handling, delivery, and other procedures used when working with Factor IX are exactly the same as described previously for Factor VIII. For more detailed information, consult the package insert or other approved literature.

CONCLUSION

You must use proper aseptic technique to prepare a sterile product, free of contaminants, ready for administration. Aseptic technique is a special skill that becomes better with experience. However, even as you begin to practice aseptic technique you must follow these guidelines, strictly, to avoid potential harm to both the patient and yourself.

PROFILES OF PRACTICE

You are working as an IV technician in the IV room alone. You get three new orders at one time—dopamine, Gammar-P IV, and a missing dose for a hydration bag. In what order should you complete these orders and why? (In most institutions any type of lifesaving drug takes precedence.)

Dopamine

1. The physician should have specified what he would like the dopamine mixed with; if it is not specified, the pharmacist needs to call and clarify. A technician may not take a verbal order. Usually dopamine is mixed with a dextrose solution.
2. Next, gather the materials needed to withdraw the dopamine and dextrose. Also, remember that since the preparation is for a neonate, all the ingredients must be preservative-free, so you need a couple of alcohol swabs and various size syringes. Remember to be as accurate as possible.
3. Calculate how much dopamine to draw up in a syringe. Using that information, determine how much dextrose you should add to correctly compound the neonatal dopamine.
4. Swab the vials and or bags and withdraw the correct amounts.
5. Depending on the institution, either call for a pharmacist check or mix the medication and then call for a check. Remember that all items compounded by a technician must be checked.
6. Does the dopamine drip go into a syringe or in an IV bag? Again, you must be familiar with the policies and procedures of the hospital. And, of course, this is a *stat* medication, which means that you have about 3 min to make it. What happens if you are wrong?

Gammar-P IV

1. Call the floor and check what time the patient actually needs this medication. This medication is very expensive and has a relatively short expiration. Conversely, if the nurse needs it now, it takes a while to make.
2. If the nurse needs the Gammar-P IV now, begin swabbing the vials and then reconstitute. While the Gammar-P IV is going into solution, make the hydration bag.

Hydration Bag

a. In order to compound the hydration bag, gather the necessary materials—usually a large-volume IV bag such as NS (normal saline or 0.9% NaCl),

KCl (potassium chloride), alcohol swabs, syringes, needles, and "Potassium Added" stickers.

b. Calculate how much KCl you should add to the IV bag.

c. Withdraw the correct amount.

d. Swab the vials and/or bags and withdraw the correct amounts.

e. Depending on the institution, either call for a pharmacist check or mix the medication and then call for a check. Remember that all items compounded by a technician must be checked.

f. Correctly label the bag. Have the pharmacist sign the label and deliver the IV bag to the floor.

3. Back to the Gammar-P IV, which is still going into solution: You might decide to help the Gammar-P IV and pick up the vial to shake it. However, before you shake the vials, remember that Gammar-P IV is a protein, and protein cannot be shaken. Shaking a protein can damage it. Instead, swirl the vial.

4. When the Gammar-P IV finally goes into solution, carefully transfer all 875 mL of the Gammar-P IV into an empty bag. Call for a check, label the Gammar, and deliver the Gammar to the floor. You are finally finished with the three new orders and can go back to finishing the regular IV pick.

This scenario could be a common occurrence at a large hospital on any given day. Can you see how any IV technician must possess proficient knowledge in such areas as medical terminology, IV room materials and supplies, different mathematical calculations, and quality assurance? There were only three orders; however, a pharmacy technician must have not only good aseptic skills, but also the knowledge needed to compound these medications correctly.

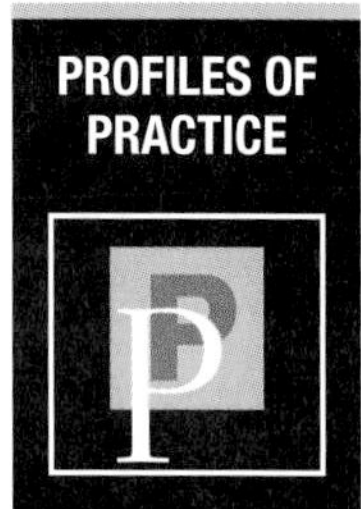

CHAPTER TERMS

immunocompromised
a condition in which the immune system is not functioning normally

reconstitute
to add a diluent to a vial to create a liquid

CHAPTER REVIEW QUESTIONS

MULTIPLE CHOICE

1. Dressing most commonly takes place in the __________.
   a. anteroom
   b. closet
   c. scrub room
   d. laboratory
   e. bathroom

2. Paper shoe covers, jackets, face masks, paper arm guards, and facial hair masks are examples of __________.
   a. TPN
   b. CCS
   c. PPE
   d. PPL
   e. DDT

3. All compounding must be performed at least __________ inside the edges of the hood.
   a. 2 ft.
   b. 8 in.
   c. 11 in.
   d. 6 in.
   e. 1 ft.

4. If the LAH has been turned off, how long must it be turned on before it can be used? __________
   a. 30 min
   b. 15 min
   c. 60 min
   d. 20 min
   e. 10 min

5. Ampules are made of __________.
   a. plastic
   b. steel
   c. polyurethane
   d. cardboard
   e. glass

6. The process of adding diluent to a powder in a container is known as __________.
   a. manipulating
   b. levigation
   c. reconstitution
   d. emulsifying
   e. additive blending

7. When withdrawing contents from an ampule, what must you use? __________
   a. lint-free towels or gauze
   b. filters
   c. 3-cc syringes
   d. transfer kit
   e. Advantage vial

8. According to ASHP guidelines, the total volume being measured must be at least __________ of the total size of the syringe.
   a. 20 percent
   b. 30 percent

c. 40 percent
d. 15 percent
e. 50 percent

9. After swabbing with alcohol, you must wait for __________ before proceeding when preparing to withdraw contents from a container with a needle/syringe.
   a. the tops to be removed from all the vials of ingredients
   b. the blower in the hood to run for at least 10 min
   c. the pharmacy technician to dress
   d. the alcohol to dry completely
   e. the IV bags to be unwrapped

10. What must you do to all vials before you bring them into the hood? __________
   a. remove the tops
   b. date them
   c. remove the labels
   d. stir them slightly to loosen the contents
   e. heat them to a lukewarm temperature

11. Why is Factor VIII gently swirled? ______________
   a. to avoid a color change
   b. to decrease the risk of precipitation
   c. so the mixture does not chemically heat up
   d. to prevent foaming
   e. to prevent cloud formations

CHAPTER 6

Sterile Product Preparations

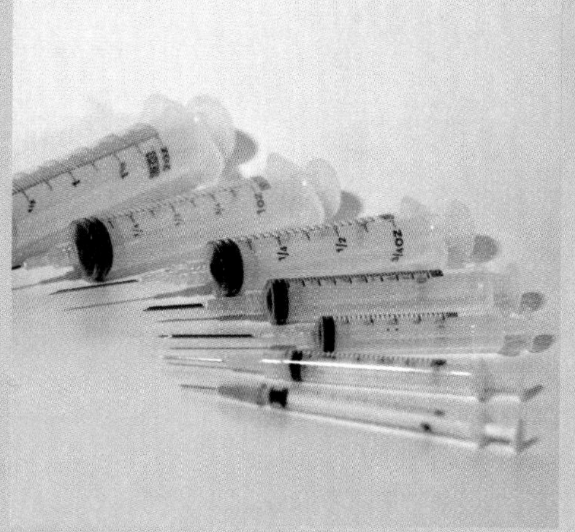

Learning Objectives

After completing this chapter, you should be able to:

- List and describe the different types of sterile products.
- Know the different uses for large-volume and small-volume IV bags.
- Understand the concept of pediatric dosing and realize why sterile products prepared for this type of patient are different from those for adults.
- List some specialty protein-based sterile products.

INTRODUCTION

There are many different ways to prepare sterile products for administration. Some medications are aseptically compounded into a syringe, whereas others are aseptically compounded into a large-volume IV bag. Other sterile medications may be in the form of irrigations or ophthalmic solutions. Most are compounded in a laminar airflow hood (LAH), whereas some are compounded in a biological safety cabinet (BSC). This chapter will explore the different ways that sterile products can be packaged for proper administration.

IV Bags

The most common type of sterile product is the IV bag. Table 6.1 displays some of the most common IV bags available and their abbreviations. IV bags contain medication that must be diluted in the IV bag before administration. For example, if Fortaz (an antibiotic) is administered IV without being diluted, it will cause a severe burning sensation to the patient. Other medications, such as potassium chloride (KCl), can cause death when undiluted.

intravenous piggyback (IVPB)
a small-volume IV fluid that normally has medication added

IV bags can be classified into two large groups. IV bags that are administered on a schedule, such as twice daily or three times a day, are referred to as **intravenous piggybacks (IVPB)** (Figures 6-1 and 6-2). The second group of IVs—large-volume IVs and drips—are usually run as a continuous preparation and generally include maintenance fluids (Figures 6-3 and 6-4). The primary distinction is between those that are scheduled and those that are run continuously.

TABLE 6-1 Infusion Fluid Abbreviations

UNSP	Unspecified
BWFI	Bacteriostatic water for injection
SWFI	Sterile water for injection
D5W	Dextrose 5% in water (5% dextrose injection, USP)
D10W	Dextrose 10% in water (10% dextrose injection, USP)
D20W	Dextrose 20% in water (20% dextrose injection, USP)
D5LR	Dextrose in lactated Ringer's solution (5% dextrose in lactated Ringer's injection)
D5$\frac{1}{4}$S	Dextrose 5% in $\frac{1}{4}$ strength saline (5% dextrose and 0.22% sodium chloride injection, USP)
D5$\frac{1}{2}$S	Dextrose 5% in $\frac{1}{2}$ strength saline (5% dextrose and 0.45% sodium chloride injection, USP)
D5NS	Dextrose 5% in normal saline (5% dextrose and 0.9% sodium chloride injection, USP)
D5R	Dextrose 5% in Ringer's injection (5% dextrose in Ringer's injection)
D10NS	Dextrose 10% in normal saline (10% dextrose and 0.9% sodium chloride injection, USP)
IS10W	Invert sugar 10% in saline (10% invert sugar in 0.9% sodium chloride injection)
LR	Lactated Ringer's injection, USP
Pr	Protein hydrolysate (protein hydrolysate injection, USP)
R	Ringer's injection, USP
NS	Sodium chloride 0.9% (normal saline) (0.9% sodium chloride injection, USP)
SOD CL 5	Sodium chloride 5% (5% sodium chloride injection)
Sod Lac	Sodium lactate, $\frac{1}{6}$ Molar (M/6 sodium lactate injection, USP)

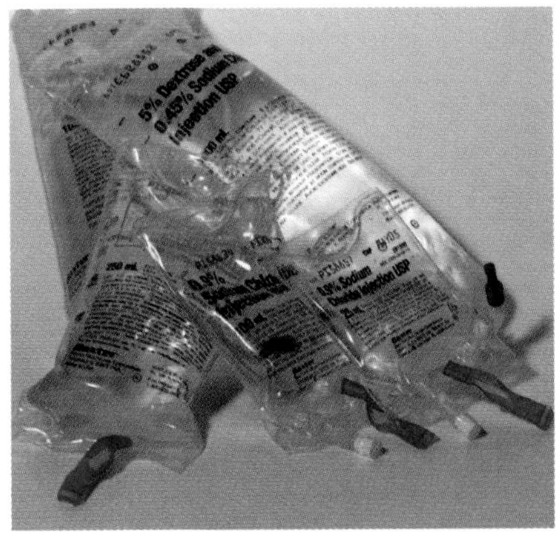

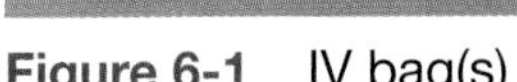

Figure 6-1 IV bag(s)

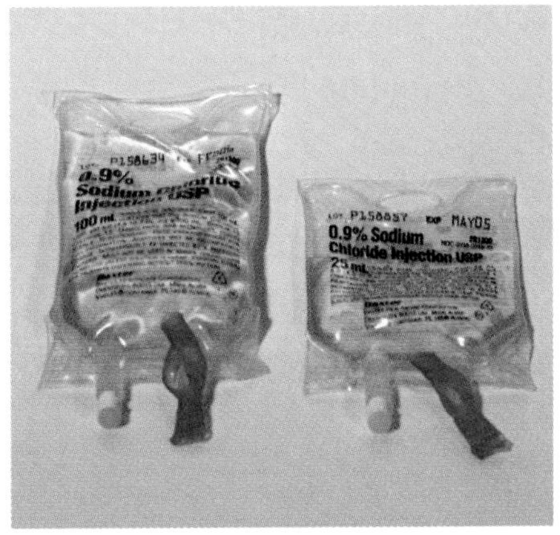

Figure 6-2 IV piggyback

IV PIGGYBACKS

Intravenous piggybacks are administered over a short period of time at certain intervals. They also usually have a smaller volume than a continuous infusion. These IVs consist of a base fluid—D5W or NS—with a medication added to the fluid.

The objective of the IVPB is to administer a medication that (1) the patient cannot take via another method or (2) needs to act quickly. These IVs are usually some type of antibiotic, antifungal, antiviral, mineral replacement, or maintenance medication. Antibiotics include, but are not limited to, Unasyn, Claforan, Fortaz, vancomycin, and Zosyn. Antivirals include, but are not limited to, Zovirax and Cytovene. Mineral replacements may include potassium chloride, sodium chloride, and calcium gluconate. Maintenance medication includes Dilantin, valproic acid, and Cerebyx.

In some hospitals, IV antibiotics are still made by reconstituting a vial and adding that vial to the base volume, creating an IVPB. Other hospitals have gone to an Add-A-Vial or Advantage system, which allows the vial to be attached aseptically in the LAH to the IV bag without mixing the contents of the vial. When the desired dose is needed, a valve in the neck of the special IV bag can be broken, allowing the contents to be mixed. The advantage to this type of system is that it has a longer expiration date than aseptically reconstituted vials, because the solutions are not mixed until just before administration. A number of IV solutions come from manufacturers premade and are kept frozen until use. Frozen IVs are mostly premade antibiotic IVPBs. The advantage to this system is that they are sterile and effective to their expiration date as long as they are kept frozen. However, once they are defrosted, they have an expiration date between 14 and 28 days. No aseptic compounding is required for this type of IVPB; they require only proper labeling and a final check by a pharmacist before delivery to the patient.

CONTINUOUS PREPARATIONS

Large-Volume IVs

Large-volume IV bags are mainly used for patients who are dehydrated and need fluid replacement. Large-volume IVs are generally 1 L; they can vary in base types depending on what the patient needs. Electrolytes and vitamins are easily added to large-volume IV bags. Often when a patient is dehydrated, vitamins and minerals are depleted as well. Large volumes can also be continuous antibiotic infusions, which are sometimes necessary to treat severe infections.

Drips

Drips are medications that are given to the patient until he shows improvement or to relieve terminal pain. Drips include nitroglycerin, insulin, amiodarone, lidocaine, Nipride, epinephrine, narcotics, and other types of emergency medication. Most hospitals have specific policies and procedures that deal with these medications because they are unusual medications and can be costly to make.

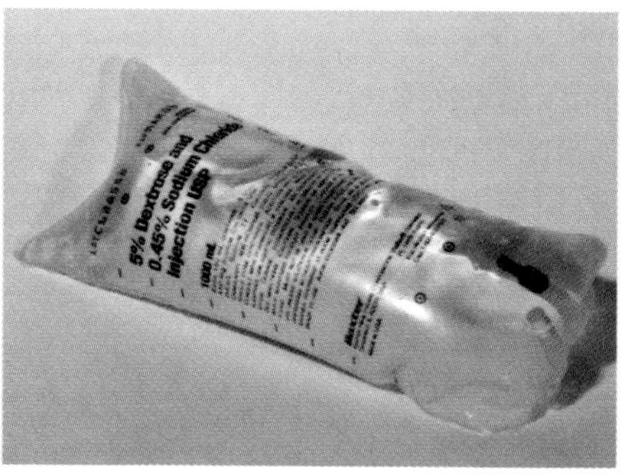

Figure 6-3 Large volume

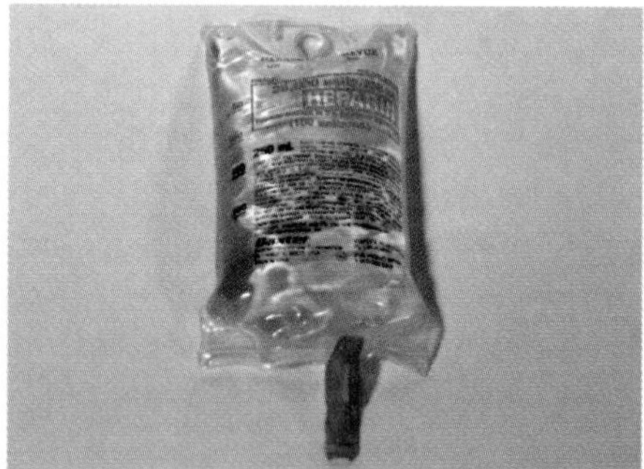

Figure 6-4 drip

Syringes

Syringes are another common form of administration used for a variety of reasons (Figure 6-5). The volume of a syringe can vary from 0.1 mL to 60 mL; if the volume of a medication can be measured in a syringe, then it can be packaged in a syringe. Some of these medications can be given without being diluted, such as skin tests, vaccinations, and epogens, whereas others such as personal controlled anesthesia (PCA), stress tests, and pediatric and neonatal antibiotics will be diluted.

Essentially, the syringe dosage form will be used for either very small amounts (skin tests, vaccinations, and epogens) or medications that must be extremely accurate (PCAs, stress tests, and pediatric and neonatal antibiotics).

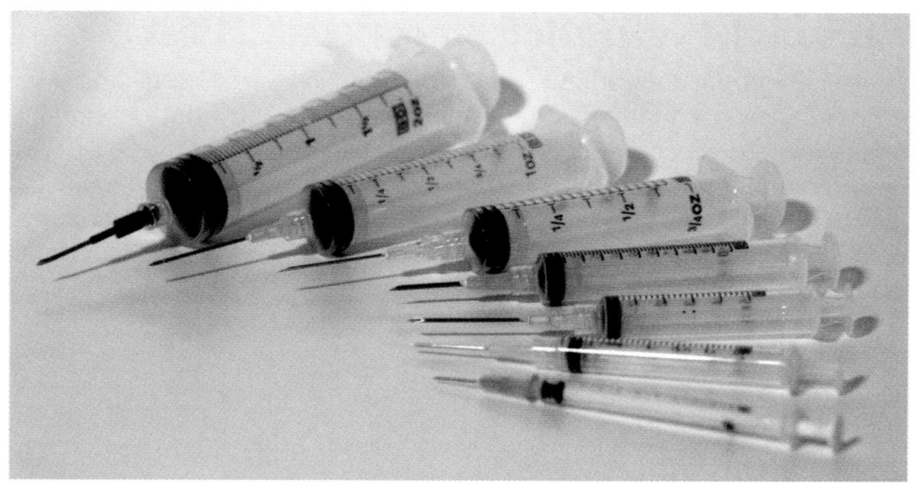

Figure 6-5 Syringes

Multidose Vials (MDVs)

In the case of skin tests, the vial is a multidose vial (Figure 6-6), which means that it can be used more than once because it contains preservatives; the amount needed for the dose is usually 0.1 mL. The dose will be administered and the remainder in the vial will be properly stored for other doses at a later time before the expiration date. This way, instead of opening a vial per dose, the pharmacy can save money by using the vial more than once, if the dose has been removed using aseptic technique and stored according to the manufacturer's requirements. The same applies to vaccinations and epogens; however, vaccination volumes may range from 0.5 mL to 1.0 mL and the epogens are based upon the dose prescribed.

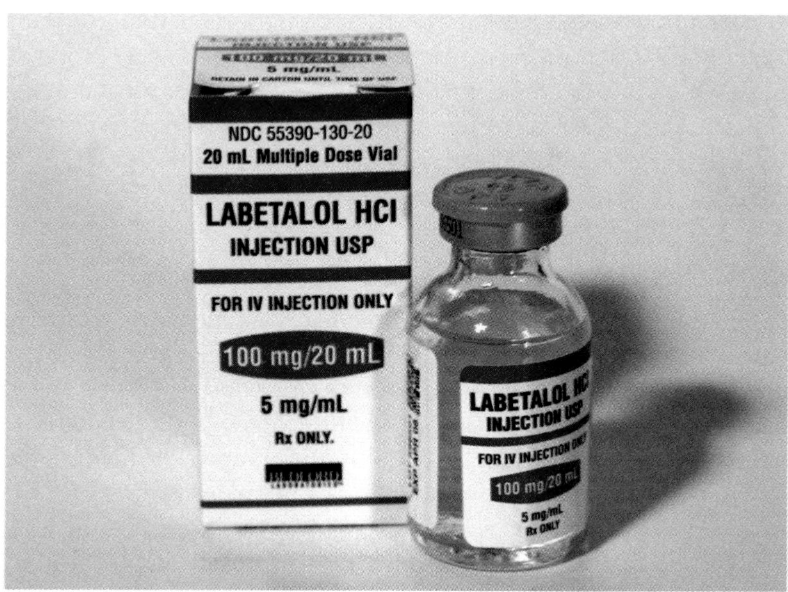

Figure 6-6 Multidose vial

Personal Controlled Anesthesia (PCA)

Personal controlled anesthesia (PCA) (Figure 6-7), stress tests, and pediatric and neonatal antibiotics and drips are cases in which the aseptic compound must be very accurate. In these cases, adding the additive to an IVPB is not accurate enough. To be as accurate as possible with small amounts, it is better to place the sterile compounds in a syringe. The other option is to entirely remove all the base fluid from an IVPB and then add only the amount of base fluid back into the IVPB.

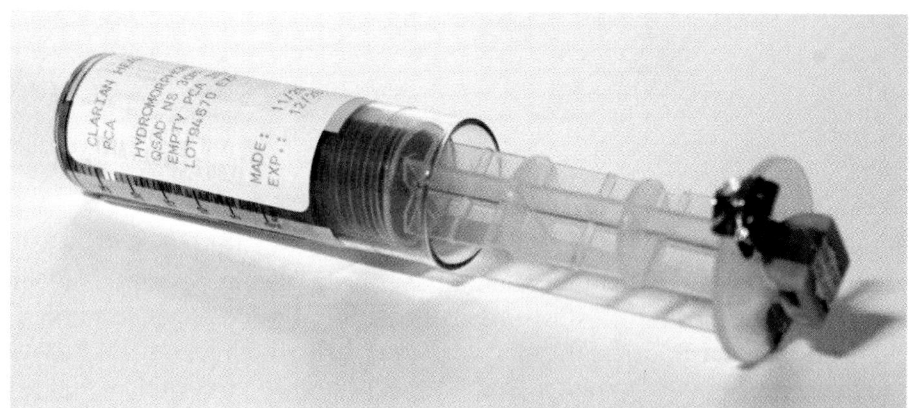

Figure 6-7 Personal controlled anesthesia

Epidurals

Epidurals are another type of dosage form that is most often used in conjunction with surgery or obstetrics (Figure 6-8). Epidurals are placed intrathecally and are used to help control pain. Epidurals may consist of a narcotic and anesthetic, such as bupivacaine or ropivacaine, or just an anesthetic, depending on the patient's needs. The important thing to remember about epidurals is that they are placed in the intrathecal space, right next to the spine, which means that all medications used to aseptically compound an epidural must be preservative-free. The most common preservative, benzyl alcohol, can cause paralysis if used in an epidural.

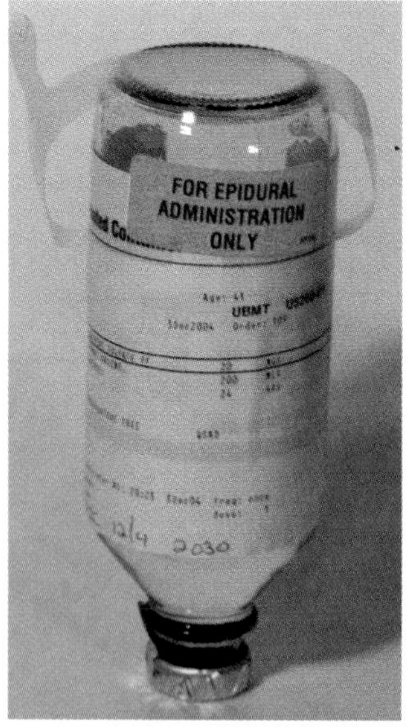

Figure 6-8 Epidural

Neonates and Pediatric Patients

Most of the time dilutions are used for neonates and pediatric patients. Dilutions are a way to take a more concentrated substance and make it less concentrated; they are usually used when a very small dose is needed and cannot accurately be measured. For example, insulin comes as 100 U/mL. The dose of insulin ordered for a neonate is 5 U. Without diluting the insulin, the dose is 0.05 mL—a very small dose. With very small amounts, it is easy to unintentionally draw up an inaccurate dose. However, if the insulin is diluted from 100 U/mL to 10 U/mL, then the same 5 U dose is now 0.5 mL, which is much easier to measure accurately.

The other reason for using dilutions is that neonatal and pediatric patients' organ systems are still developing. Their liver and kidneys do not metabolize and excrete medications as efficiently as those of most adults. Diluting the medication, or putting the dose in a larger fluid amount, is less taxing on the developing systems. Most medications can be made into dilutions. These medications include, but are not limited to, antibiotics, antifungals, antivirals, narcotics, and insulin.

Irrigations

Irrigations also may be compounded aseptically (Figure 6-9). The most common sterile irrigations are surgical antibiotic solution (SAS) and gentamicin irrigation solution. These are not true aseptic compounds, but these irrigations must be compounded in a sterile environment. They are typically used in surgery to irrigate open surgical sites. The bottles or IV bags to which Neosporin and gentamicin are added are sterile. They have a label that states "Sterile Water (or Saline) for Irrigation Only." This means that the solutions are sterile but do not meet the requirements to be used intravenously.

irrigation
a solution used for washing

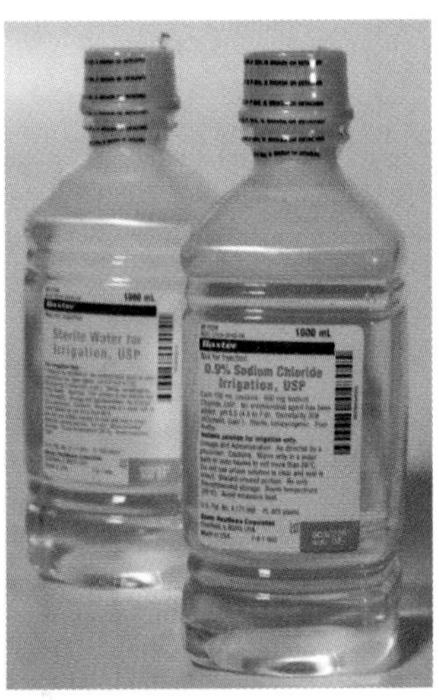

Figure 6-9 Irrigation

Cytotoxic Agents

Cytotoxic (chemotherapy) medications are always compounded in a biological safety cabinet (BSC) (Figure 6-10). The BSC has a different direction of airflow (vertical) that allows the IV technician to compound cytotoxic medications more safely. Instead of flowing toward the IV technician, the air is blown vertically down; this way the aerosols produced when making the cytotoxic compound are not blown toward the IV technician. Chemotherapy medications come in a variety of forms: syringes, IVPBs, or continuous infusions. The only difference between cytotoxic medications and other dangerous drugs is where they are aseptically compounded.

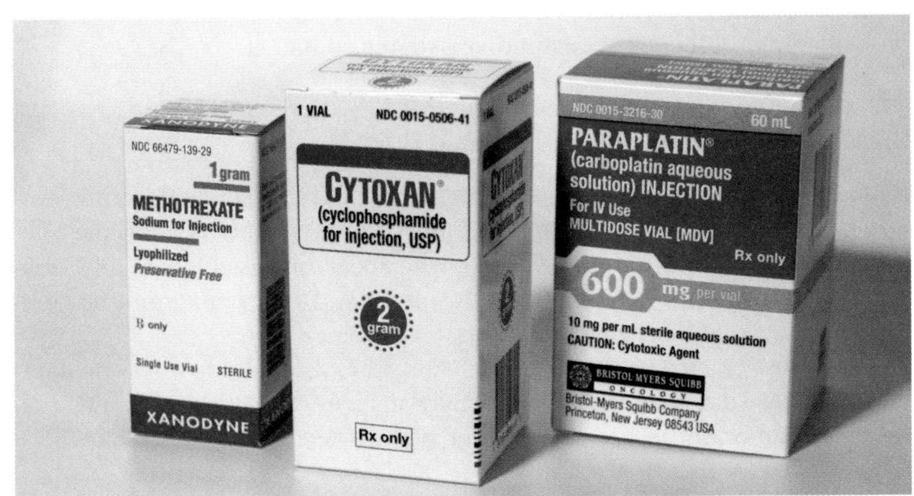

Figure 6-10 Cytotoxic agents

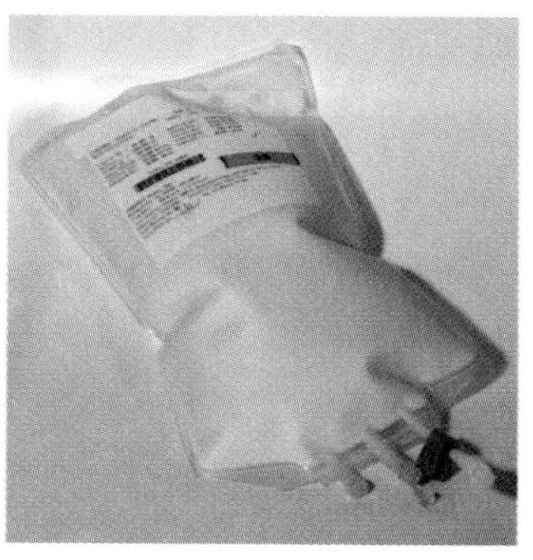

Figure 6-11 TPN bag

Total Parenteral Nutrition (TPN)

A physician may decide to order a total parenteral nutrition (TPN) bag (Figure 6-11) if a patient has not been able to receive adequate nutrition via other means. TPNs are essentially a meal in intravenous form. They can contain proteins, fats, sugars, water, minerals, electrolytes, and vitamins. TPNs are compounded daily, usually every 24 hr, specific to the patient's needs and size, and may range in size from 500 mL to 3000 mL.

Proteins

Special preparations are also an important part of the aseptic compounding in an IV room. Most of these special preparations are proteins. They should never be filtered as they will stick to the filter, thus altering the dose given.

ALBUMIN

Some of the special preparations are albumin, plasma protein fraction, Gammar, Factor VIII, and Factor IX. Albumin is a sterile solution for a single-dose administration, containing 25% human albumin. Albumin is used to treat hypovolemic shock, in conjunction with exchange transfusion, in the treatment of neonatal hyperbilirubinemia, and for other conditions. Albumin may be a floor stock item in critical-care areas. Do not use albumin solutions if they appear turbid or if there is sediment in the bottle. Begin administration within 4 hr after the bottle is punctured. Dispose of empty albumin vials in an approved sharps container.

PLASMA PROTEIN FRACTION (PPF)

PPF is a sterile solution for single-dose intravenous administration containing 5% plasma proteins. PPF is used to prevent and treat hypovolemic shock and cases of severe hypoproteinuria, as in adjunct hemodialysis. Do not use solutions of PPF if they appear turbid or if there is sediment in the bottle. Begin administration within 4 hr after the container has been entered. Dispose of empty PPF vials in an approved sharps container.

IMMUNOGLOBULIN (GAMMAR, IgG)

Immune globulin intravenous is a sterile, lyophilized, single-dose preparation of immune globulin. Gammar is indicated for patients with primary defective or suppressed immune systems, who are at increased risk of infection. Wear chemo gloves when preparing this product. Do not mix immune globulin products of differing formulations.

IgG must be reconstituted before being administered. Most IgG preparations include a double-ended, vented spike adapter with a plastic piercing pin. It is very important to use the transfer pins correctly. Failure to follow the reconstitution instructions could lead to contamination of the product and/or loss of vacuum, which would make IgG impossible to reconstitute. Read the package insert for step-by-step reconstitution instructions. Do not shake the product vial, as excessive foaming and protein bruising will occur. Gently swirl the vial once the diluent has been added. Use within 24 hr of reconstitution, or as recommended by the package insert. Visually inspect the solution for any particulate matter and discoloration prior to administration. Dispose of empty IgG containers, tubings, and so on in an approved sharps container. Check with the pharmacy's policies and procedures before compounding any IgG, as Gammar has a short stability time and is very expensive.

FACTOR VIII (ALPHANATE)

Factor VIII is a sterile, lyophilized, single-dose concentrate of antihemophilic factor (AHF). Factor VIII is used to prevent and control bleeding in patients with Factor VIII deficiency due to hemophilia-A or acquired Factor VIII deficiency. Wear chemo gloves when preparing this product. Do not mix Factor VIII products from differing formulations.

Factor VIII is ordered in units; lyophilized Factor VIII concentrate is available in many different sizes. The number of units in the vial varies with each lot number. When preparing Factor VIII, try to come as close as possible to the number of units that the physician orders. If it is impossible to get the exact number of units ordered, always go over; never go under the amount of units that the physician orders.

Always draw up the complete vial; never use a partial vial in an attempt to get an exact dose. Label the dose with the exact amount contained in the syringe. Factor VIII is usually stored in the refrigerator (some brands are stored in the freezer); whenever possible, remove the Factor VIII from the refrigerator approximately 30 min before reconstitution. This allows the concentrate and the diluent to warm to room temperature and helps the concentrate dissolve more easily. Reconstitute the concentrate according to the package insert instructions. Do not shake the reconstituted product, as excessive foaming will result. Gently swirl the contents once the diluent has been added. Withdraw the reconstituted product into a syringe through the vented filter spike provided in the package. Whenever possible, do not fill the syringe to more than two-thirds of its maximum capacity.

Before capping with a red leur-lock syringe cap, draw approximately 10 cc of air into the syringe. This will reduce bubbling and foaming and, more important, will reduce the risk of exposure to nursing staff if the AHF leaks into the cap or the transport bag. Administer Factor VIII within 8 hr or as directed in the package insert. Discard all empty AHF vials and associated tubing, equipment, and so on into an approved sharps container.

Check with the pharmacy's policies and procedures before compounding any scheduled doses of Factor VIII, since this product has a short stability, is extremely expensive, and is very unlikely to be able to be used on another patient.

FACTOR IX (KONYNE)

Factor IX is a sterile, lyophilized, single-dose concentrate of AHF intended for IV administration to treat Factor IX deficiency. The reconstitution, handling, delivery, and other procedures used when working with Factor IX are exactly the same as described previously for Factor VIII. For more detailed information, consult the package insert or other approved literature (Figure 6-12).

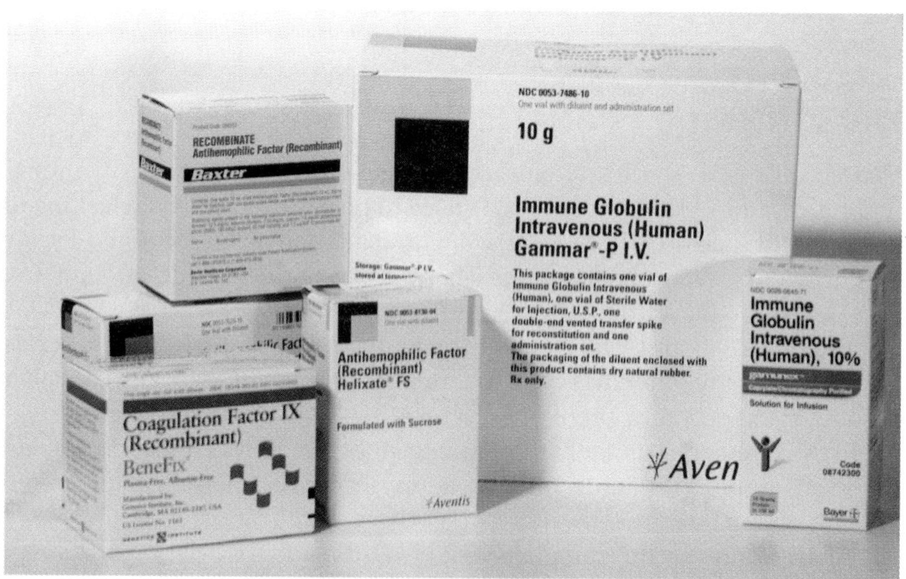

Figure 6-12 Special protein products

Ophthalmics

Ophthalmics must be sterile because when an eyedrop is placed in the eye, it is readily absorbed (Figure 6-13). In most cases, the pharmacy purchases sterile ophthalmics, but in some institutional pharmacies or specialty pharmacies, physicians will request a specific ophthalmic preparation that cannot be purchased. In those cases, the ophthalmic preparation must be aseptically prepared. Each ingredient must be filtered, which is a method of sterilization.

These medications are aseptically compounded in a laminar airflow hood and then autoclaved, which is the process of subjecting a compound to immense heat. The compound is sterilized by the heating or autoclaving process. The ophthalmic preparation is then cultured to ensure that the solution contains no possible contaminants. The entire process can vary from 7 to 14 days.

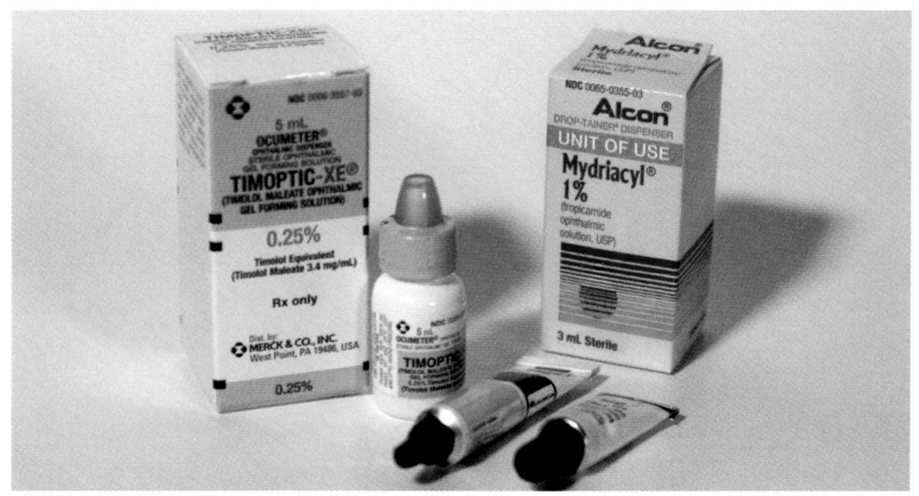

Figure 6-13 Ophthalmic preparation

CONCLUSION

A wide variety of dosage forms are used in conjunction with sterile products, depending on the desired route of administration. The most common route of administration that requires aseptic preparation is intravenous. The IV route of administration involves a large number of potential dosage forms, including syringes, IVPBs, drips, and large-volume IV bags. With experience you will learn not only how a specific product is made, but also the best method of preparation.

CHAPTER TERMS

intravenous piggyback (IVPB)
a small-volume IV fluid that normally has medication added

irrigation
a solution used for washing

CHAPTER REVIEW QUESTIONS

MULTIPLE CHOICE

1. Which is the most common form of IV administration? __________
   a. syringes
   b. IV bags
   c. epidurals
   d. ophthalmics

2. What is the most common way that IV antibiotics are compounded? __________
   a. large volumes
   b. syringes
   c. intravenous piggybacks
   d. irrigations

3. A physician writes an order for a TB skin test. How should this request be made? __________
   a. syringe
   b. IVPB
   c. large volume
   d. send up the bottle and the nurse can draw up the test

4. A physician writes an order for a neonatal dopamine order. The total volume must be 50 mL. What should the dosage form be?
   ____
   a. syringe
   b. IVPB
   c. large volume
   d. intrathecal

5. A physician writes an order for a D5NS 1-L bag to be infused at 125 mL/hr for 24 hr. What type of dosage form should be used? __________
   a. syringe
   b. IVPB
   c. large volume
   d. send up the bottle and the nurse can draw up the test

6. A physician writes an order for an epidural that has fentanyl and bupivacaine in normal saline. Which of the following statements is incorrect?
   ____
   a. The IV technician should take into account the total size of the epidural.
   b. The IV technician should never put narcotics in an epidural.
   c. The IV technician should never put preservatives in an epidural.
   d. The IV technician must use aseptic technique.

7. A __________ vial allows the medication in the IV bag to be mixed just before administration.
   a. last-minute-adding
   b. Micromix
   c. Advantage
   d. epidural
   e. none of the above

8. PCA stands for __________.
   a. patient comfort anesthesia
   b. piggyback chemical additives
   c. partially combined additives
   d. piggyback combined anesthesia
   e. personal controlled anesthesia

9. Surgical antibiotic solution (SAS) is an example of a sterile compounded __________.
   a. irrigation
   b. epidural
   c. PCA
   d. IV piggyback
   e. drip

10. Factor VIII should be removed from the refrigerator at least __________ before administering.
   a. 15 min
   b. 60 min
   c. 45 min
   d. 20 min
   e. 30 min

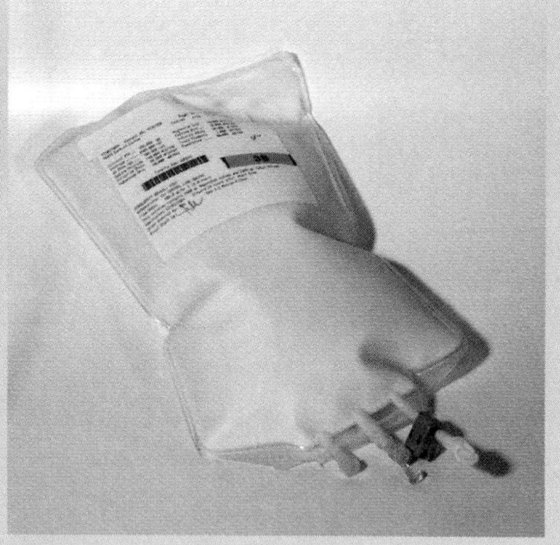

CHAPTER 7

Total Parenteral Nutrition (TPN)

Learning Objectives

After completing this chapter, you should be able to:

- Explain why a patient receives a TPN.
- List the additives used in making a TPN.
- Explain why the ingredients are necessary in a TPN.
- Describe how to admix a TPN.
- Discuss automated mixing equipment.

INTRODUCTION

Total parenteral nutrition (TPN) provides an alternate nutritional route in cases of severe gastrointestinal distress and/or poor nutrient absorption. TPNs are given to patients who cannot or should not receive their nutrition through eating. They are prescribed by a physician to meet a person's entire nutritional needs. TPNs nourish the body and relieve the digestive tract while therapy for the underlying condition progresses.

TPN IV bags can also be called hyperalimentation bags (hyperals). They provide protein, lipids, sugar, electrolytes or salts, vitamins, and other essential elements. This liquid food substitute is infused directly into a vein, typically over 10–12 hr. The IV route can be through a central line or a peripheral line.

A patient may require a TPN for any of several reasons. A TPN may be given to a patient who:

- has cancer
- has AIDS
- has Crohn's disease

- has had surgical removal of the intestines
- has severe diarrhea
- has hyperemesis gravidarum (uncontrollable vomiting during pregnancy)
- is a premature **neonate**
- is in a coma

neonate
a newborn baby

The Ingredients

These sterile compounds may have up to 15–20 additives, which make them extremely complex. The more complex, the higher incidence of error or incompatibility. A TPN is made between the range of 500 mL to 4 L, with the average being 3–4 L unless it is prescribed for a child. Because of the nature of the ingredients, perfect aseptic technique must be maintained to reduce the possibility of contamination while compounding a TPN. For example, lipids help provide a fertile medium for the growth of microorganisms. Since TPNs are administered directly into the bloodstream, sepsis is a major concern.

As previously mentioned, TPNs contain a myriad of essential ingredients all necessary to human functions, including the following:

- sugar (such as dextrose for energy)
- carbohydrates (for energy)
- protein (for muscle strength)
- lipids (fat)
- electrolytes (such as sodium, potassium, chloride, phosphate, calcium, and magnesium)
- amino acids (a source of nitrogen)
- trace elements (such as zinc, copper, manganese, and chromium)

A TPN order may contain all or some of these substances, depending on the patient's condition. Everyone needs these base ingredients in addition to other substances to stay healthy.

The following is a list of TPN additives that may be used:

Base Components:

Amino acids 10%, trophamine 6%
Dextrose 70%, dextrose 50%
Sterile water
Lipids 20%

Additives:

Sodium acetate
Sodium chloride
Sodium phosphate
Potassium acetate

Potassium chloride
Potassium phosphate
Magnesium sulfate
Calcium gluconate
Heparin
Zinc
Insulin
Trace elements
Chromium
Copper
Multivitamin for injection
Insulin
Pepcid
Zantac

FLUID MAINTENANCE

The physician will begin by deciding the total volume of the TPN and choosing the base fluid. A first estimate of maintenance fluid requirements can be obtained from body weight or from body surface area. The figure based on body weight is obtained from the following mathematical formula:

100 mL/kg for the first 10 kg of body weight
\+ 50 mL/kg for the next 10 kg of body weight
\+ 20 mL/kg for each kilogram over 20
___
Total fluid requirement

Factors that can affect these amounts include dehydration, overhydration, and related conditions. Patients are monitored for fluid balance variations as well as nutritional needs.

CALORIES AND CARBOHYDRATES

Although caloric sources such as fructose and sorbitol have been used in TPNs, the most common sources of calories and carbohydrates are dextrose and fat. Dextrose is available in a wide range of concentrations, from 2.5 to 70%. Most commonly, 50–70% is used for TPN mixtures. Each gram of dextrose in these solutions provides 3.45 kcal.

Lipids are added to prevent essential fatty acid deficiency and in combination with dextrose to contribute to the total caloric content. Lipids are available in concentrations of 10%, 20%, and 30%. The 10% or 20% concentrations may be infused directly into the vein, while the 30% concentration is admixed into the TPN solution. This is because the osmolarity and pH balance of body fluids are more compatible with the 10% and 20% than with the 30%. It is estimated that an average, healthy patient's caloric support is best provided as a mixed fuel, with 50–80% of the calories derived from dextrose and 20–50% from fat. Each gram of fat provides approximately 9 kcal.

AMINO ACIDS AND NITROGEN

Amino acids are the molecular units that make up proteins. They are considered the building blocks of the body, as they aid in many bodily functions. Along with other essential and nonessential proteins, amino acids help provide enough nitrogen for the patient. Nitrogen levels need to be monitored and maintained, and they can vary based on different stress situations with the patient. Nitrogen aids in the protein handling of the body.

ELECTROLYTES AND MINERALS

Each patient is assessed and the physician prescribes the correct amount of electrolytes and minerals based on the patient's needs. It is extremely important that TPN orders continue to be reassessed, as the patient's needs vary daily with therapy. These additives are calculated to provide a proper balance within the body. The amounts must be accurately determined to prevent metabolic disturbances and other serious health consequences due to one or more deficiencies.

Table 7.1 presents average daily electrolyte and mineral requirements and their function during intravenous feeding. In addition to the ingredients shown in Table 7.1, injectable trace elements are added to the admixture. Vitamin K may also be mixed into the solution on a weekly basis.

TABLE 7-1 Daily Electrolyte and Mineral Requirements

Substance	Daily Requirement	Use
Sodium	80–100 mEq/day	Determines total body water May be added as chloride, lactate, acetate, or phosphate salt
Potassium	80–100 mEq/day	Contributes to proper nerve and muscle function (including the heart); regulates the water balance of cells; balances electrolytes May be added as chloride, phosphate, or acetate salt
Chloride	Usually equal to sodium	Helps keep the amount of fluid inside and outside cells in balance; helps maintain proper blood volume, blood pressure, and pH of body fluids. To avoid acid-base disturbances due to chloride ion abnormalities, the infused sodium:chloride ratio should be adjusted to 1 : 1 by using acetate, lactate, or phosphate salts instead of chloride
Calcium	15–20 mEq (0.2–0.3 mEq/kg/day)	Necessary for many normal functions of the body, especially bone formation and maintenance—nerve function, muscle contraction, blood clotting, and proper heart function Given as gluconate, glucoheptonate, or gluceptate salt
Magnesium	15–25 mEq (0.25–0.35 mEq/kg/day)	Important for many systems in the body, especially the muscles and nerves Given as magnesium sulfate
Phosphate	20–30 mM (7–9 mM/1000 kcal)	Needed for bone growth, energy, fighting infection, and proper muscle function Given as potassium or sodium phosphate

The Order

The life cycle of a TPN order begins with the physician. After assessing the patient and determining that a TPN is necessary, a physician will write the order and send it to the pharmacy to be compounded. Most facilities that compound TPN solutions will have written **protocols** for the management of TPN. Patients are assessed daily and appropriate changes are made based on the clinical course of the patient and available laboratory data.

protocol
the standard plan for a course of medical treatment

The hospital pharmacy may have a *standard order*, which is the basic, nonspecialized TPN order for an average TPN patient, as part of its protocol, or the physician can deviate from the standard order and create his own specialized TPN order. Each order will consider whether the TPN is to be administered though a **central line** or a **peripheral line**. Factors considered when deciding on a peripheral or central line include the following:

central line
a larger blood vessel

peripheral line
a small vein in the hand, foot, or head

- type of medication being administered
- osmolarity and pH of the solution to be infused
- duration of therapy
- diagnosis or medical condition of the patient
- patient preferences
- current availability and status of patient's veins
- patient history
- secondary risk factors

There may be other factors to consider as well. Each patient is assessed as an individual.

Hypertonic mixtures of amino acids and dextrose may be safely administered by continuous infusion through a central line. For patients for whom a central line is not indicated, a peripheral line may be used with a diluted dextrose 5–10% solution prepared as an isotonic or slightly hypertonic solution.

It is important to infuse the TPN solution at a steady rate. Large changes can result in significant **hypoglycemia** or **hyperglycemia**. Sometimes infusion is interrupted for different reasons. A bag of low-concentration dextrose, such as 5%, can be infused during the interruption to help prevent sudden hypoglycemia caused by the high endogenous insulin secretion associated with the infusion of hypertonic dextrose.

hyperglycemia
too high a level of glucose

hypoglycemia
too low a level of glucose

Compounding the TPN

When the pharmacy receives a TPN order, the pharmacist or CPhT checks the patient's lab values. The pharmacist then compares the lab values to the TPN order and suggests any clinical changes if necessary. The pharmacist also goes over the calcium gluconate and potassium phosphate levels to help ensure that the TPN will not precipitate. Phosphate supplementation is often incompatible with calcium, which causes the formation of an insoluble salt.

After checking the levels, either the pharmacist or a CPhT performs the calculations necessary to determine how a TPN will physically be made. In order words, if the order is written for 6 mEq KCl per liter and the total actual volume

(TAV) is 1.5 L, then 9 mEq needs to be added to the TPN ($6 \times 1.5 = 9$). If KCl comes as 2 mEq/mL, this means that 4.5 mL of KCl must be added to the TPN $\left(\frac{9}{2} = 4.5\right)$. After all the calculations are complete, a pharmacist must double-check them. Some hospitals require two pharmacists to check the TPN calculations before preparing the TPN. It is very easy to make mistakes when dealing with TPNs, as they are very complex. Great detail and care must be exercised.

After the TPN calculations are completed and double-checked, it is time to compound the TPN. TPNs are usually compounded in a laminar airflow hood (LAH), but may be compounded in a biological safety cabinet (BSC) if a LAH is not available.

The TPN is broken down into two main sections—the base and the additives. The base, which is composed of dextrose, amino acids, sterile water for injection (SWFI), and sometimes lipids, makes up the majority of the volume of the TPN. Additives make up the other part. Additives include electrolytes, vitamins, minerals, and whatever else the physician has ordered to make the TPN patient-specific. The number of different additives can range from 5 to 20, with an average of 10 to 25 different ingredients.

Some institutions that compound large numbers of TPNs may have some automated devices to help, such as an Automix. These devices can calculate the amount of each additive needed for the TPN, yet still require some input of data. They can also pump the correct amount of fluid into a TPN bag based on the *specific gravity* (discussed later). Other institutions that either compound small numbers of TPNs or do not regularly compound TPNs may compound the entire TPN by hand.

After dressing and washing your hands, gather all the supplies and ingredients necessary to compound the TPN. Carefully check the amounts needed for each ingredient and choose the correct size bags, syringes, and needles. For example, if 6 mL of a product is needed, then choose the next higher syringe, 10 mL, for drawing up that particular ingredient. To choose a bag, calculate the final volume of the TPN and use a bag in which the entire TPN will fit easily. It is better to choose a bag that is too big than one that is not big enough.

After you check the base components, inject them into an empty IV bag, also called a Viaflex bag, using a male adapter or a port adapter. The port adapter can be used for injection several times while making only one injection into the TPN bag. This way the TPN bag injection port is not compromised. Add the base components to the TPN bag in the following order: dextrose, amino acids, lipids (if present), and SWFI. Do not add the lipids until the end, because the mixture is opaque white and will prevent visual inspection for precipitates and other particulates in the solution. The amino acids act as a buffer between the dextrose and lipids to minimize any possible chemical reaction.

In many compounding areas, transfer bags and kits are available. Transfer kits include tubing used to transfer fluid from one container to another. For example, you would use a tranfer kit to transfer large volumes of dextrose into a much larger bag, as it would be quite time-consuming to draw out 1 L using a 60-mL syringe.

It is extremely important for the pharmacy technician to learn what supplies are available for compounding and what procedures are followed. Some

WORKPLACE WISDOM

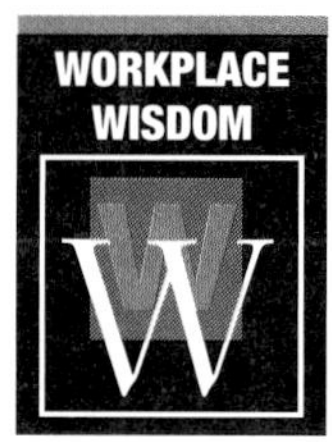

Check with the hospital's policies and procedures to see if syringes are uniformly placed on the right or left side of the vial. Whatever the pharmacy decides, it should remain consistent to help prevent medication errors. Remember, it is very difficult to determine what is in a clear, unmarked syringe. When in doubt, toss it out.

supplies make compounding easier, reducing manipulations, whereas other facilities may not have such supplies and would require more steps in the procedure and more safety precautions. Know what supplies are on hand and know how to use them.

After the large-volume fluids are admixed, excluding the lipids, begin drawing up the individual ingredients in individual syringes. Make sure that each aseptic manipulation is done in a clean air space. Most TPNs have many different additives to be withdrawn and space can become constricted. After you withdraw the additives, place the syringes right next to the vial you drew them from.

After you draw up the additives, the pharmacist must perform a final check. After the final check is complete, inject the additive syringes into the TPN bag. When adding additives to a TPN, there is no set order; the potassium phosphate is added first, the calcium gluconate is added second to last, and the multivitamin for injection (MVI) is added last. Make sure to gently mix the bag in between the addition of the additives. Potassium phosphate and calcium gluconate can cause precipitation to occur in a TPN if they are added too closely together. The MVI is added last so that any precipitation is not masked. If you add any proteins such as insulin or albumin to the TPN, remove any filters that were used because the proteins will stick to the filters altering the dose.

Be sure to add any lipids last. Lipids, as previously mentioned, are a solid milky white liquid that will mask any particulate or precipitation in the final solution. When you have finished admixing all ingredients, gently shake or rotate the bag to blend and distribute the ingredients evenly.

When you add the calcium at the end of the admix procedure and again when you have finished adding all ingredients, be certain to carefully inspect the solution visually. Take time to survey closely and notice any particulates. If you find any, notify the pharmacist immediately.

Before delivering the solution to the patient, some facilities will include an inline filter. There is some debate over the usefulness of such filters and whether they are necessary. One concern is that they may clog the additives, such as the fat emulsions. Check with the facility and its procedures to see if a filter is included with TPN solutions.

Automated Devices

Automated devices include automix, micromix, and the gravity method.

AUTOMIX

Clinitec has developed TPN software that can control the automated TPN Automix compounder. The Automix compounder is linked to a computer that controls how much is pumped into a TPN bag. First, the physician writes a TPN order that goes to the pharmacy. The pharmacist or CPhT enters this information into the Clinitec computer, which then calculates how much of each ingredient is to be added. The computer displays warnings if any of the preprogrammed levels are off, including any precipitation problems. Then a label is printed out and checked by another pharmacist, or possibly two.

After the labels are checked, the technician programs the Automix compounder for the correct patient, hangs the correct size bag, and then pushes the Start button. The Automix compounder begins to push the fluid out of the base component bags into the TPN bag, which hangs on a hook that actually weighs the TPN bag as it is being pumped.

The compounder uses each base component's **specific gravity** to pump the correct amount into the TPN bag. For example, amino acids have a specific gravity of 1.07 mg/mL. If the total amount of amino acids needed in the TPN is 84 mL, we multiply 84 × 1.07 = 89.88 mg. After the Automix compounder measures that amount of amino acid, it automatically moves on to the next solution that needs to be pumped into the IV bag. As a safety feature, the Automix compounder also gives an alarm if a solution does not have the same specific gravity for which it is programmed. For example, if a bag of SWFI is hung (specific gravity 1.00) instead of a bag of dextrose 70% (specific gravity 1.24), then the machine would give an alarm to inform the user that the specific gravities do not match, which would indicate a medication error.

specific gravity
the weight of a substance compared (as a ratio) with that of an equal volume of water

MICROMIX

The newest automated device is the Micromix compounder, and pharmacies are just starting to acquire them. The Micromix compounder can add up to ten additives to the TPN bag. This significantly reduces the amount of syringes that must be drawn for each TPN. As long as the computer has been correctly programmed, the error rate is reduced. The Micromix compounder adds the additives to the TPN bag using the specific gravity of each additive. It works similarly to the Automix compounder, but with greater accuracy.

The Micromix compounder can pump as little as 2 mL correctly into a TPN bag and can measure to tenths (0.1 mL). The Micromix compounder is designed to add medications in the order programmed and to flush the lines between the different additives. Even though the Micromix compounder can add up to ten additives, the IV technician usually still must pull a couple of additives by hand. These additional additives should be aseptically withdrawn and placed in a clean air space near the TPN with the vial from which they were drawn.

GRAVITY METHOD

Not all facilities use automated admixture machines. The gravity method is used to prepare some IV admixtures without such equipment. In this method, one additive is placed higher than the other (typically one is hung from a pole in the hood or BSC) to produce a continuous free flow.

CONCLUSION

Certain patients in institutional settings must receive their daily nutrition from a TPN. These orders must be precise and can become quite complicated, due to the sheer number of ingredients or additives involved. While some facilities now use automated technology to aid in the preparation of TPN orders, you must still be competent in this area if you will be using such equipment.

PROFILES OF PRACTICE

TPNs are considered an acute treatment, one with a specific length of duration, in most cases. Controversy has risen, however, as some physicians use TPNs to extend the life of a small number of children born with nonexistent or severely birth-deformed intestines. The oldest of these patients turned 8 years old in 2003.

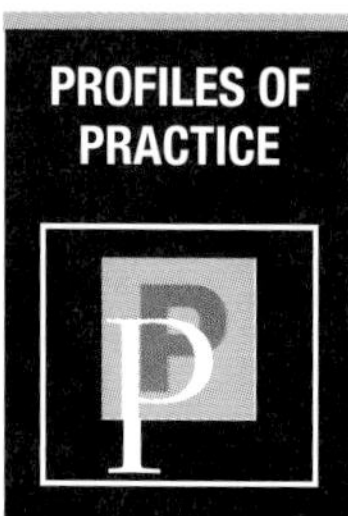

CHAPTER TERMS

central line
a larger blood vessel

hyperglycemia
too high a level of glucose

hypoglycemia
too low a level of glucose

neonate
a newborn baby

peripheral line
a small vein in the hand, foot, or head

protocol
the standard plan for a course of medical treatment

specific gravity
the weight of a substance compared (as a ratio) with that of an equal volume of water

CHAPTER 7

CHAPTER REVIEW QUESTIONS

MULTIPLE CHOICE

1. What does TPN stand for?
   a. total purchasable nutrition
   b. total parenteral naturalism
   c. total parenteral nutrition
   d. the parenteral nutrition
   e. total parental nutrition

2. What is not another name for TPN? __________
   a. the food bag
   b. total parenteral nutrition
   c. hyperalimentation bag
   d. hyperal
   e. bag

3. What two additives should never be mixed closely together? __________
   a. potassium chloride and potassium phosphate
   b. potassium chloride and calcium gluconate
   c. calcium gluconate and potassium chloride
   d. potassium phosphate and calcium gluconate
   e. calcium chloride and magnesium sulfate

4. In a hospital, who is responsible for writing a TPN? __________
   a. IV technicians
   b. pharmacists
   c. nurses
   d. physicians
   e. nurse practitioners

5. In a hospital, who is responsible for making clinical changes to a TPN? __________
   a. IV technicians
   b. pharmacists
   c. nurses
   d. physicians
   e. pharmacy residents

6. Which of the following patients is a possible candidate for a TPN? __________
   a. a cancer patient
   b. a neonatal patient
   c. a surgical patient
   d. a pregnant patient
   e. all of the above

7. Where is a TPN typically compounded? __________
   a. by the patient's bedside
   b. in a laminar airflow hood
   c. in a biological safety cabinet
   d. in a pharmacy
   e. in the outpatient pharmacy

8. What additive should be added last to a TPN? __________
   a. potassium chloride
   b. potassium phosphates
   c. calcium gluconate
   d. multivitamin for injection
   e. dextrose

MATCHING

Please indicate whether each item is an additive or a base component. Put the appropriate letter by the additive or the base. Answers may be used more than once.

9. __________ sterile water
10. __________ sodium acetate
11. __________ sodium chloride
12. __________ sodium phosphate
13. __________ TrophAmine 6%
14. __________ potassium acetate
15. __________ potassium chloride
16. __________ dextrose 70%
17. __________ potassium phosphate
18. __________ magnesium sulfate
19. __________ calcium gluconate
20. __________ amino acids 10%
21. __________ heparin
22. __________ zinc
23. __________ trace elements
24. __________ chromium
25. __________ lipids 20%
26. __________ copper
27. __________ multivitamin for injection
28. __________ insulin
29. __________ dextrose 50%
30. __________ Pepcid

a. additive
b. base component

Chemotherapy

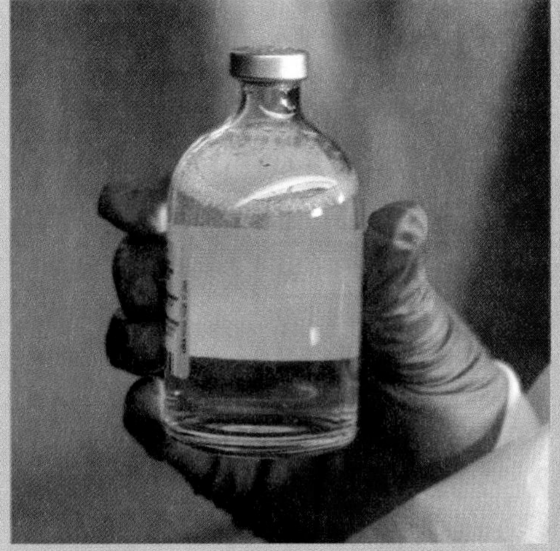

Learning Objectives

After completing this chapter, you should be able to:

- Describe what happens with cancer and cells.
- Explain how cytotoxic agents are used to treat cancer.
- Explain safety procedures for handling chemotherapy agents.
- Describe types of biological safety cabinets.
- Discuss appropriate procedures for preparing chemotherapy agents.
- List the hazards involved with preparing chemo agents.
- Describe how to clean a chemo spill.

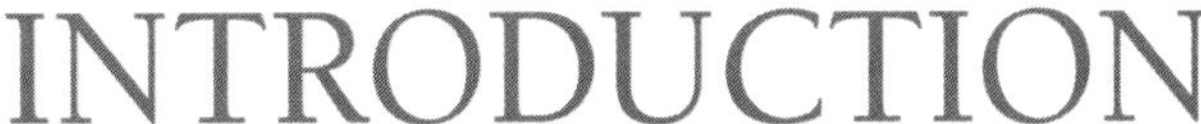

INTRODUCTION

Cancer is a difficult disease. Cancer cells develop because of damage to DNA that causes cells in a part of the body to begin to grow out of control. Most cancers produce tumors, but some, such as leukemia, do not. Various types of cancer behave differently, grow at different rates, and respond to different treatments. This is why they require treatment that is specific to the cancer type. The earlier a cancer is found and treatment begins, the better the chances for survival. The treatment for cancer is also difficult. There are many different types of cancer; the treatment may range from removing the **malignant** cells to **chemotherapy** and radiation.

malignant
tending to become progressively worse and to result in death

chemotherapy
treatment of cancer with drugs (chemicals)

The following is a partial list of types of cancer:

Bladder cancer
Bone cancer
Brain cancer
Breast cancer
Cervical cancer
Colon cancer
Esophageal cancer
Extrahepatic bile duct cancer
Gallbladder cancer
Hodgkin's disease
Kidney cancer
Laryngeal cancer
Leukemia
Liver cancer
Lung cancer
Lymphoma
Melanoma
Multiple myeloma
Oral cancer
Ovarian cancer
Pancreatic cancer
Pharyngeal cancer
Prostate cancer
Rectal cancer
Skin cancer
Stomach cancer
Testicular cancer
Uterine cancer
Vaginal cancer
Vulvar cancer

Several viruses are also known to be linked to cancer:

- Long-standing liver infection with the hepatitis virus can lead to cancer of the liver.
- A variety of the herpes virus, the Epstein-Barr virus, causes infectious mononucleosis and has been implicated in non-Hodgkin's lymphomas and nasopharyngeal cancer.
- The human immunodeficiency virus (HIV) is associated with an increased risk of developing several cancers, especially Kaposi's sarcoma and non-Hodgkin's lymphoma.
- Human papilloma viruses (HPVs) have been linked to cancers of the cervix, vulva, and penis.

Although cancer is one of the primary reasons a patient will receive chemotherapy treatment, it is not the only reason. Chemotherapy may also be used to treat rheumatoid arthritis, lupus, psoriasis, and other autoimmune diseases. Our focus, however, will follow suit with aseptic preparation in the IV realm, which is typically used for patients with cancer.

The general idea of chemotherapy is to kill the tumor or the malignant cells without causing more damage than necessary to the patient. There is no cure for cancer, yet treatment with potent medications such as cytotoxic agents and antineoplastics can often suppress symptoms and provide better quality of life for the patient.

Some cancer types tend to affect a certain population more than others. For example, children tend to be diagnosed with leukemia, while women get breast, ovarian, and uterine cancer; men are more at risk for prostate and colon cancer and smokers have a higher incidence of lung cancer. Other cancers affect populations uniformly, such as brain tumors, liver cancer, and kidney cancer.

With a significant amount of the population being diagnosed with cancer, compounding **cytotoxic** agents is becoming a more common practice. This chapter is designed to help IV technicians protect themselves while also providing the best possible care for the patient.

cytotoxic
describes chemicals that are directly toxic to cells, preventing their reproduction or growth

Cytotoxic Agents

Cytotoxic agents, or **antineoplastics**, are generally used for patients with various forms of cancer. These types of drugs are extremely toxic to cells. Many chemotherapy medications are indicated for specific tumors or cells. The idea behind cytotoxic drugs is to kill the cancer or tumor without killing the patient. Unfortunately, chemotherapeutic agents cannot tell the difference between a healthy cell and a sick cell. This is why some patients succeed in eliminating the cancer but also have unwanted side effects such as hair loss.

antineoplastic
a drug intended to inhibit or prevent the maturation and proliferation of neoplasms that may become malignant

Generally speaking, there are two classes of antineoplastic agents:

Cycle-Phase-Nonspecific Agents—These agents work on a cell at any time during the cell's cycle. There are five main types:

- Nitrogen mustards
- Ethylenimines
- Alkyl sulfonates
- Triazenes
- Nitrosoureas

Cycle-Phase-Specific Agents—These agents work on a specific cycle during the cell (most are nonresting). These agents are indicated for rapidly growing tumors where there is a high growth period. Antimetabolites are most commonly used for these types of tumors. Some examples are etoposide, hydroxyurea, vincristine, and vinblastine.

Take care when working with all antineoplastic agents, as they are potentially mutagenic (can cause cells to mutate), **carcinogenic** (can cause cancer), **teratogenic** (can cause birth defects), and immunosuppressive.

carcinogenic
producing a malignant new growth that arises from the epithelium, which is found in skin or, more commonly, the lining of body organs

teratogenic
tending to produce anomalies of formation

The following is a list of some common cytotoxic medications that the IV technician may come across:

Asparaginase (Elspar)
Bleomycin (Blenoxane)
Carboplatin (Paraplatin)
Carmustine (BiCNU)
Cisplatin (Platinol)
Cladribine (Leustatin)
Cyclophosphamide (Cytoxan, Neosar)
Dacarbazine (DTIC-Dome)
Dactinomycin (Actinomycin)

Daunorubicin (Cerubidine)
Doxorubicin (Adriamycin, Doxil, Rubex, hydroxydaunomycin, hydroxydoxorubicin)
Estramustine (Estracyt)
Etoposide (VePesid, Etopophos)
Floxuridine (FUDR, fluorodeoxyuridine)
Fluorouracil (5FU)
Gemcitabine (Gemzar)
Idarubicin (Idamycin)
Ifosfamide (Ifex)
Mesna (Mesnex)
Methotrexate (MTX, Amethopterin)
Mitomycin (Mytomycin-C, Mutamycin)
Paclitaxel (Taxol)
Plicamycin (Mithramycin)
Rituximab (Rituxan)
Thiotepa (Thioplex)
Vidarabine (Vira-A)
Vinblastine (Velban)
Vincristine (Vincasar, Oncovin)

Compounding Chemotherapy Medications

Compounding chemotherapy medications is a useful skill for any technician who would like to work in an IV room. When performed properly, this task is no more dangerous than compounding other sterile products. It is important to remember, however, that cytotoxic agents are toxic and are deadly to cells. The risks are great if these products come into contact with human skin. Mixing chemotherapeutic agents requires a strict degree of carefulness, to avoid harm to the personnel preparing these products.

As with most medication orders, the physician initiates a chemotherapy drug order (Figure 8-1). The order is then sent to the pharmacy, where the pharmacist double-checks the order to ensure that it is written correctly. Then the IV technician begins to gather the necessary materials to compound the chemotherapy medication.

15246
CH-69
(JUN 02)

013105

ADULT PARENTERAL NUTRITION ORDER

03/11/1944 F 12/27/04

TRANSPLANT
INPATIENT

A. Check INDICATION for Parenteral Nutrition

☐ Bowel Ischemia
☐ IDB/short bowel syndrome
☐ Intractable Vomiting/Diarrhea
☐ Gi Bowel Obstruction/Teus
☐ Fistula
☐ Other ________

B. BASE SOLUTION

☐ **CUSTOM CENTRAL FORMULA**

1. Protein
   Crystalline Amino Acids 60 g/days
   Hepatamine* (40 g/bottle) ____ g/days
2. Nonprotein Calories (NPC)
   Dextrose 1000 kcal/day
   Fat 300 kcal/day
3. Total volume (check one)
   ☐ a. Maximally concentrated solution
   ☒ b. 1800 mL/day

☐ **STANDARD CENTRAL FORMULA** (per liter)

Amino Acids	50g
Dextrose	600 kcal (175g)
Fat	300 kcal (30g)
Total kcal	1100 kcal/L
Total Volume ________	mL/day

☐ **STANDARD PERIPHERAL FORMULA** (per liter)

Amino Acids	30g
Dextrose	240 kcal (70g)
Fat	400 kcal (40g)
Total kcal	760 kcal/L
Osmolarity	710 mOsm/L
Total Volume ________	mL/day

C. ADDITIVES (Guidelines for electrolytes/vitamins on back)

☐ **CUSTOM**		☐ **STANDARD**	
Sodium Acetate	40 mEq/day	Sodium Phosphate	20 mE/day
Potassium Chloride	40 mEq/day	Magnesium Sulfate	12 mEq/day
Potassium Phosphate	____ mEq/day	Multivitamin	10 mEq/day
Calcium Gluconate	5 mEq/day	Insulin (Humulin R)	____ units/day
Multi-Trace Elements	1 mL/day		

D. METABOLIC MONITORING Check box if desired. (Enter I.U. Order No. in parenthesis.)

☐ Chem 7 qd or q ____ ( )
☐ Ionized Ca. Phos. Mg q. Monday/Thusday ( )
☐ Prealbumin every Monday ( )
☐ Glucose monitoring q 6 hours or q ____ ( )
☐ Hepatic Panel and Triglycerides q Monday ( )
☐ Weigh patient qd or q ____ ( )

Special Instructions: ________

Physician Signature: ________ Date 1/31/05 Time 13,30

RN/Unit Secretary Signature: ________ Date ____ Time ____

WHITE-MED. RECORD
CANARY-PHARMACY

ADULT PARENTERAL NUTRITION ORDERS **T-5**

B.-CLIN. NOTES	E-LAB	G-X-RAY	K-DIAGNOSTIC	M-SURGERY	Q-THERAPY	T-ORDERS	W-NURSING	Y-MISC.

Figure 8-1 Chemo order

PREPARATION AREAS

biological safety cabinet (BSC)
a type of airflow hood in which chemotherapy drugs are compounded

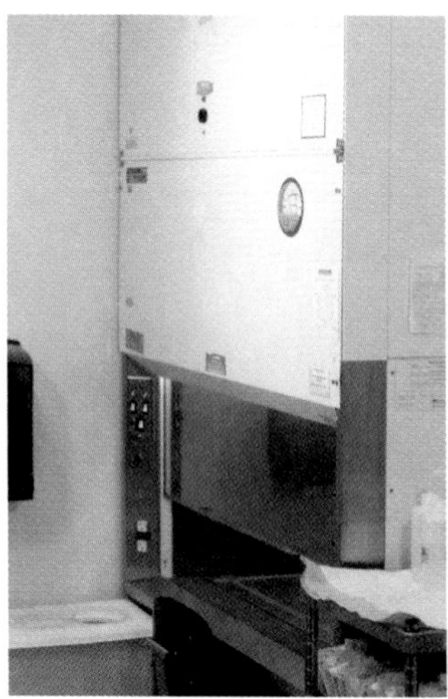

Figure 8-2 BSC

chemo mat
an absorbent mat used in the BSC over which the IV tech should compound cytotoxic agents so any spills can be absorbed

Facilities that compound chemotherapeutic agents are subjected to at least the same stringent requirements for the clean room atmosphere where the mixing of regular IVs takes place. There are necessary additions, however, such as biohazard waste containers, spill kits, special gloves, shower apparatus, dispensing pins, and other related supplies. Again, it is very important that you become familiar with USP 797 guidelines and keep up to date with any revisions; these guidelines also apply to chemotherapeutic preparations.

Biological Safety Cabinets

Chemotherapy medications are compounded in a **biological safety cabinet (BSC)** (Figure 8-2), similar to the LAH. BSCs are also known as vertical airflow hoods. BSCs are designed to provide personnel, product, and environmental protection when proper procedures are followed.

A chemotherapy mat (also called a **chemo mat** or diaper) is placed inside the biological safety cabinet (BSC) to absorb any leaks or spills. The same sterile materials used in the IV hood may also be used in the BSC.

There are several types of biological safety cabinets. BSCs are available in Class 1, 2, or 3. Table 8.1 lists the differences according to risk assessment. Chemotherapy agents should be prepared in a Class II BSC, which is a vertical airflow cabinet containing high-efficiency particulate air (HEPA) filters.

The main difference between BSCs is that some are vented directly to the outside and others filter the air again before circulating it back into the clean room air. This type of hood has a front glass cover (view screen) that is brought down when mixing to leave a 6-in. opening to enter and work through.

- The *Class I BSC* provides personnel and environmental protection, but no product protection. It is similar in air movement to a chemical fume hood, but has a HEPA filter in the exhaust system to protect the environment.
- The *Class II BSC* provides personnel, environmental, and product protection. Airflow is drawn from around the operator into the front grille of the cabinet, which provides personnel protection. In addition, the downward laminar flow of HEPA-filtered air provides product protection by minimizing the chance of cross-contamination along the work surface of the cabinet.
- The *Class III BSC* was designed for work with biosafety level 4 microbiological agents and provides maximum protection to the environment and the worker. It is a gas-tight enclosure with a non-opening view window.

These BSCs work great depending on how many and what types of chemo agents are being compounded in the clean room. For institutions that do not compound cytotoxic agents on a regular basis, a BSC that recirculates the filtered air back into the room will suffice. However, if ten or more cytotoxic agents are being compounded weekly, then a BSC that vents directly to the outside is preferred.

TABLE 8-1 Comparison of BSC Characteristics

BSC Class	Face Velocity	Airflow Pattern	Applications	
			Nonvolatile Toxic Chemicals and Radionuclides	Volatile Toxic Chemicals and Radionuclides
I	75	In at front; exhausted through HEPA to the outside or into the room through HEPA	Yes	Yes (1)
II, A	75	70% recirculated to the cabinet work area through HEPA; 30% balance can be exhausted through HEPA back into the room or to the outside through a thimble unit	Yes	No
II, B1	100	Exhaust cabinet air must pass through a dedicated duct to the outside through a HEPA filter	Yes	Yes (minute amounts (2))
II, B2	100	No recirculation; total exhaust to the outside through hard duct and a HEPA filter	Yes	Yes (small amounts)
II, B3	100	Same as II, A, but plenums are under negative pressure to room; exhaust air is thimble-ducted to the outside through a HEPA filter	Yes	Yes (minute amounts (2))
III	N/A	Supply air inlets and hard duct exhausted to outside through two HEPA filters in series	Yes	Yes (small amounts)

BSCs must be validated for integrity at least every six months. The HEPA filter must be recertified every six months or if the hood is moved, since relocating a BSC may break the HEPA filter seals or otherwise damage the filters or the cabinet.

BSCs blow clean air from the top of the hood vertically toward the bottom of the hood, unlike the laminar airflow hood, which blows clean air horizontally toward the IV technician. With this vertical flow of air, the cytotoxic fumes are kept in the hood. The IV technician must always keep the direction of the airflow in mind to prevent **shadowing**. Shadowing occurs when airflow in the BSC is blocked.

shadowing
the act of blocking airflow in the BSC

Glove Box Isolators

The glove box isolator type of BSC is a specially designed airflow hood that helps restrict free movement of contaminants. It is a contained unit in which the operator slips his hands into long glovelike parts whose surface is completely encompassed inside the hood. This type of hood is highly favored by USP 797 guidelines as appropriate for use in multitasking situations. Glove box isolators requires less space, have monitoring controls, and are basically self-contained.

Proper Use of the BSC

The BSC requires the same consideration as the LAH while in operation. Some key points to keep in mind are as follows:

- Keep the insides and tops of BSCs free of unnecessary equipment or supplies.
- Turn off all UV lights whenever the laboratory is occupied.
- Wash hands and arms with germicidal soap before and after work in the BSC.
- Wear a long-sleeved gown with tight-fitting cuffs and surgical gloves as part of your PPE.
- Do not eat, drink, apply cosmetics or lip balm, store food, or smoke in the laboratory.
- Dispose of sharps in a puncture-resistant container. Do not resheath or remove used needles; insert the whole assembly into the container.
- Clean up spills immediately.
- Properly dispose of all waste materials into biohazard containers.
- Disinfect interior surfaces of the work area using freshly prepared 70% isopropyl alcohol or another appropriate disinfectant.
- Place everything you need for the complete procedure in the cabinet before starting work and limit passing in or out through the air barrier until the procedure is completed.
- Set the view screen at the proper height.
- Wait 5 min after you have placed all materials in the BSC before beginning work. This will enable the BSC to purge airborne contaminants from the work area.
- Work as far to the back of the BSC workspace as possible.
- Do not work in a BSC while a warning light or alarm is signaling.
- After you complete your work, enclose or cover all equipment and materials. Allow the BSC to run for 5 min to purge airborne contaminants from the work area.
- Periodically decontaminate under work grills and work surfaces if these parts are removable.
- When the blower is shut off, the air barrier is destroyed. Within seconds, the inside of the cabinet becomes contaminated with microorganisms from the laboratory. For this reason, the BSC is generally operated with the blower turned on 24 hr a day.

Preparing to Use the Hood

1. Turn off ultraviolet light as soon as you enter the room.
2. Check the flow alarm system audio and visual alarm function (if so equipped).
3. Decontaminate readily accessible interior surfaces with a disinfectant appropriate for the agents or suspected agents present and wait at least 10 min.

As you are now aware, frequent cleaning is paramount in clean room settings. The following is a basic procedure you can use. Facilities may have slight variations, but the basic procedure is universally acceptable.

Cleaning and Decontaminating the BSC (Figure 8-3)

1. Dress for cytotoxic drug preparation.
2. Wash your hands thoroughly with a germicidal cleanser.
3. Use a clean, lint-free cloth in the following steps.
4. Keeping in mind the direction of the airflow, begin cleaning the bar at the top of the hood.
5. Then move to the back panel of the hood. Begin cleaning at the top of the panel in a side-to-side motion, working toward the bottom.
6. Move to the side panels and begin cleaning them the same way as the back panel.
7. Clean the work surface area. Start at the back of the work surface area, cleaning side to side, working toward the front of the hood.
8. Leaving the blower on in the hood, begin scrubbing from top to bottom with the cleaner. Rinse with deionized water.
9. Repeat this process with 70% isopropyl alcohol.
10. Leave all movable parts inside of the hood. Remove nothing from the hood. Only clean and move items to the side so that you can clean other parts.
11. Clean heavily contaminated areas, such as a spillage trough, twice.

Shutting Down the BSC

1. Decontaminate all items in the interior work area and readily accessible interior surfaces with a disinfectant appropriate for the agents or suspected agents present, them remove them.
2. Turn on ultraviolet light.
3. Allow 5 min of operation to purge the system. Then wait at least 10 min.
4. Turn off the BSC blower if your facility has this procedure.

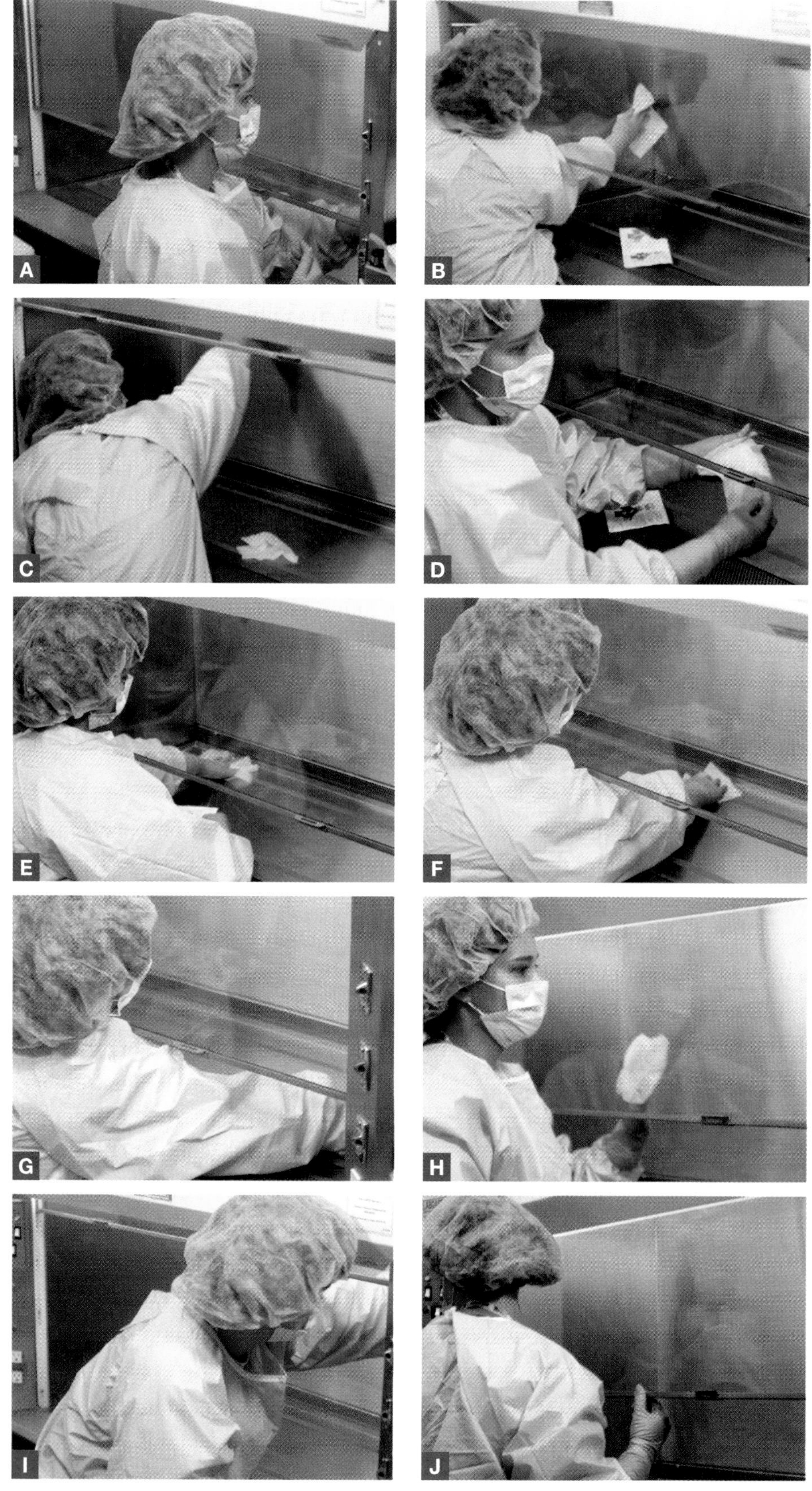

Figure 8-3 Cleaning the BSC

PERSONNEL TRAINING

It is extremely important to properly train personnel who will be mixing chemotherapy products and assess their competency prior to mixing. Competency should be assessed at least annually. Highly skilled, trained employees are essential for safety in the chemotherapy process. As part of the training program, it is highly recommended to review and test employees for competency to ensure that they have been adequately trained. Proper training, competency assessment, and ongoing education regarding chemotherapy preparation cannot be emphasized enough for the pharmacy technician working in this area.

A good training program should include a certification course that requires recertification on a regular basis, such as yearly. The trainer of such programs should, at a minimum, have several years of experience and be quite knowledgeable with chemo drugs as well as with other related information regarding chemotherapy preparation.

Chemotherapy preparation is an ongoing, complex process with changes occurring constantly. This field also requires knowledge of related information such as chemo procurement, storage, safe handling procedures, and preparation and waste guidelines for chemotherapy procedures. Up-to-date information relating to chemo preparation, policies, procedures, regulations, drugs, and other topics should be accessible to personnel at all times and maintained by the workplace.

ATTIRE

Unlike other types of sterile products, compounding chemotherapy drugs requires specific attire (Figure 8-4). In addition to the sterile cap and shoe covers, the IV technician must also wear a lint-free gown, goggles, and gloves. The additional gowning attire is designed to protect the IV technician in a worst-case scenario. Many chemotherapy drugs are irritants; acute side effects from skin exposure include skin irritation, blistering, and discoloration.

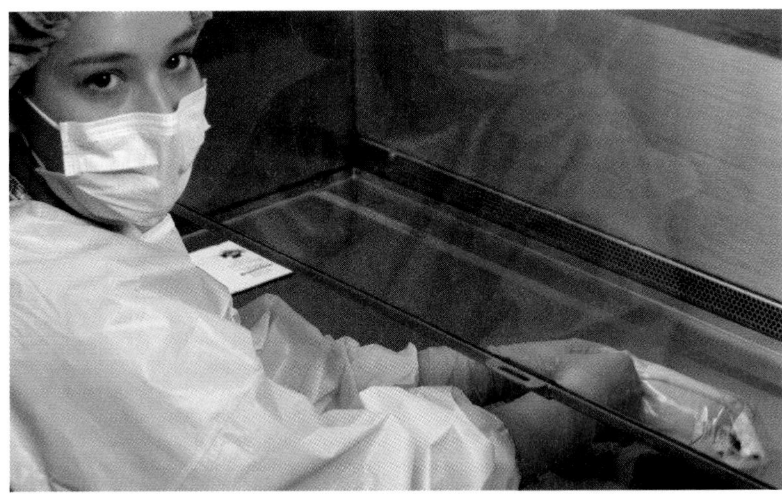

Figure 8-4 Chemo attire

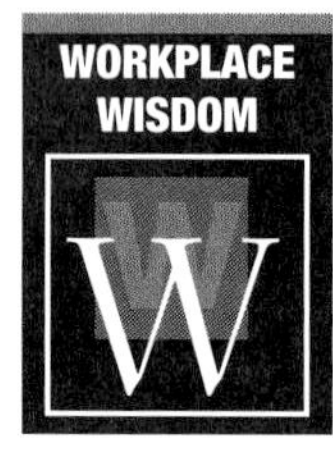

When you have brought materials into the BSC, do not bring them out again. You can leave them in the BSC until you use them, or dispose of them in the **yellow hazardous disposal container**. But do not put them back into the regular stock.

yellow hazardous disposal containers containers used to dispose of hazardous medications and the equipment used to compound them; these containers require special disposal

aerosolization suspension of small particles (liquid or powder) in the air

The following are some guidelines for chemo attire:

- When gowning up for a chemo, use a low-permeability, solid-front gown that ties in the back.
- Wear disposable, high-cuff, latex or nitrile gloves when working with biohazards (latex gloves are permeable to organic solvents).
- Use the thickest gloves allowed by your workplace to protect against cuts and scratches without compromising dexterity.
- Wear two pairs of thinner gloves to permit safe removal of the outer pair in case of inadvertent contamination.
- Wear a disposable lab coat, closed and with the sleeves tucked into the gloves, while in the lab.
- Do not wear lab coats outside the laboratory.
- Wear eye protection, such as goggles provided by your workplace.

Withdrawing a Cytotoxic Agent

You must perform this procedure using proper aseptic technique (Figure 8-5):

1. Gather all materials needed for the manipulation.
2. Most important, remember the direction of the airflow. In the BSC the air flows downward. In order to manipulate items aseptically, you must not block the airflow. In other words, do not place your hands or fingers between items that must remain sterile and the direction of the airflow.
3. Swab the rubber top with alcohol. Allow the alcohol to dry.
4. Ensure that the needle is firmly attached to a leur-lock syringe.
5. Pull the plunger back on the syringe to approximately half the amount of drug needed.
6. Never put a volume of air into the vial that is greater than or equal to the desired amount of cytotoxic agent that you need to withdraw. This will cause positive pressure in the bottle, creating **aerosolization** of the cytotoxic agent.
7. Remove the cap from the needle. Find the center of the stopper and insert the needle, bevel end up.
8. Turn the vial on its side so that clean air can blow directly on the sterile parts of the syringe and stopper.
9. Holding the syringe on the bottom side, so as not to disrupt airflow, slowly add the air from the syringe into the vial. In some cases, it may be necessary to add the air 1 mL at a time.
10. Remove the desired amount of cytotoxic agent by pulling back on the plunger.
11. When the desired amount is reached, remove the needle from the vial.
12. Remove any air bubbles using an empty evacuated container.
13. Recap the syringe.
14. Perform a final check.

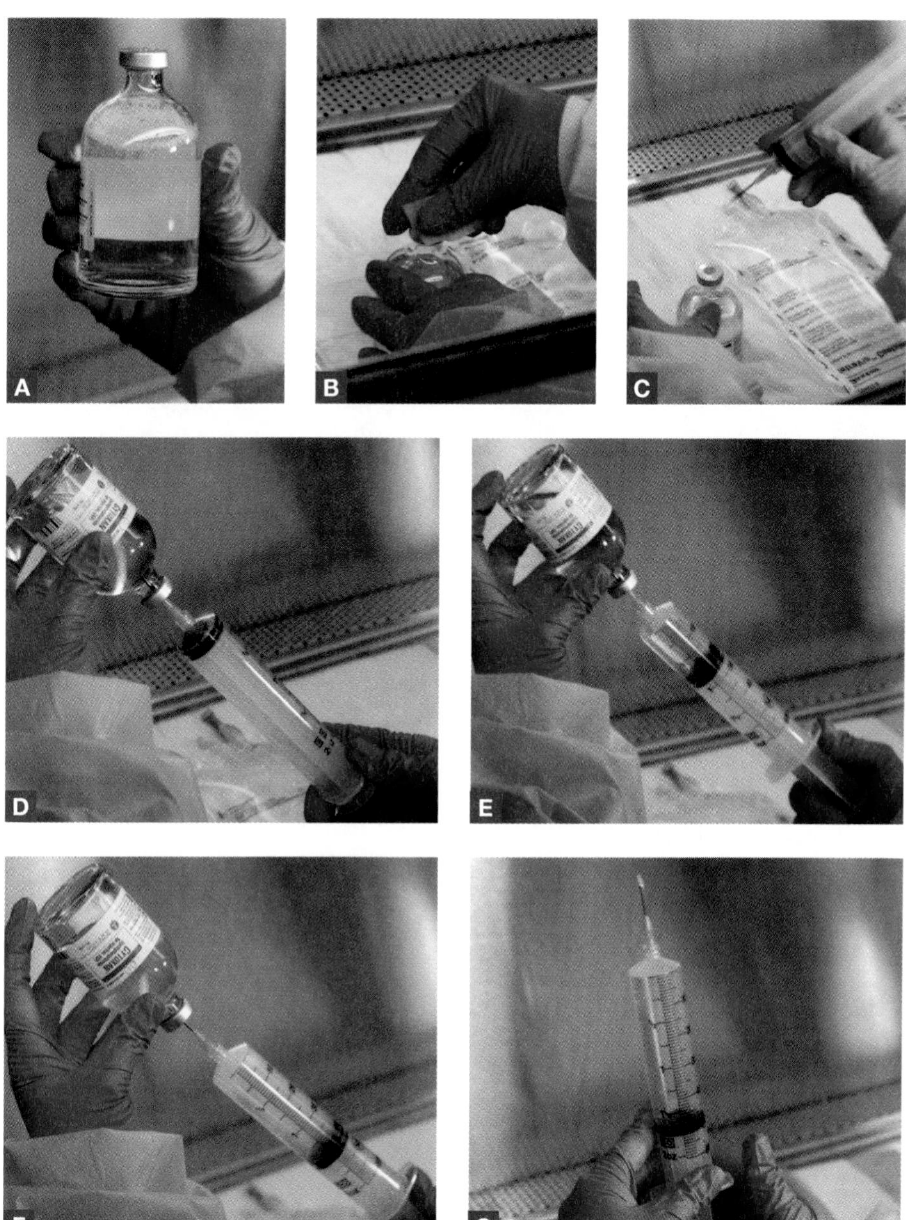

Figure 8-5 Withdrawing a cytotoxic agent

Procedures for Handling Sterile Injectable Hazardous Drugs

This section is very important, so please make sure to read it carefully.

- Ensure that syringes and IV sets have leur-to-leur connections (Figure 8-6).
- Do not fill syringes more than three-quarters full to prevent accidental separation of the plunger (Figure 8-7).
- Use venting devices with 0.2-micron hydrophobic filters and 5-micron filter needles/straws for additional protection (Figure 8-8).
- Do not use ordinary vented needles.
- Dispense final products in a ready-to-administer form.

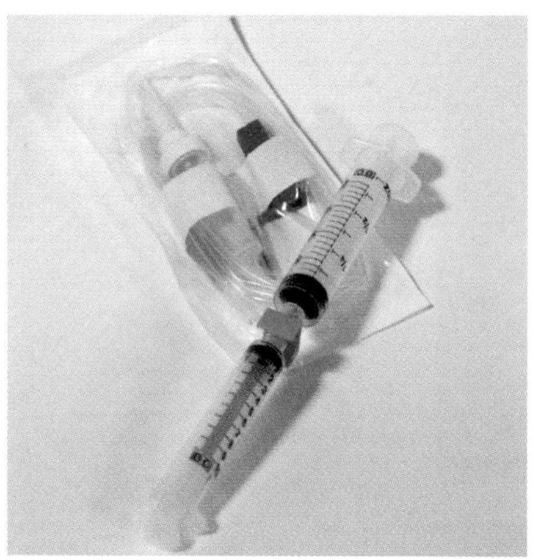

Figure 8-6 Luer-to-Luer syringe and IV set

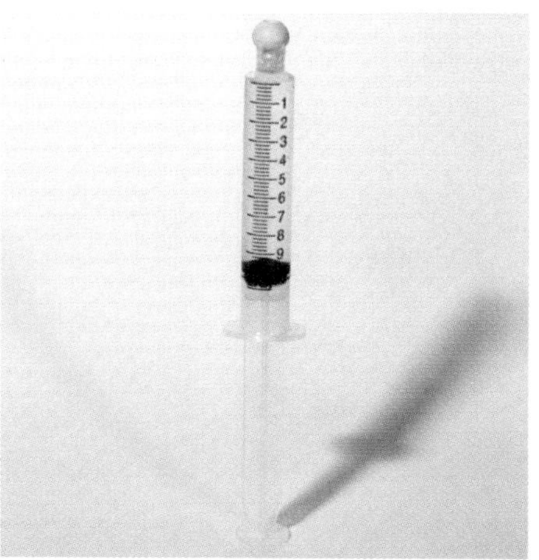

Figure 8-7 Properly filled syringe

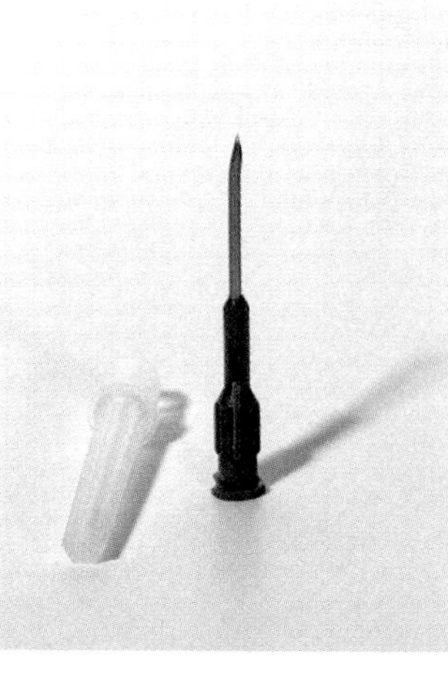

Figure 8-8 Venting devices

- Wipe the outsides of containers and IV sets with moist gauze to remove any inadvertent contamination. Also wipe all IV ports clean and cover them with a foil cap (Figure 8-9).
- Label final products, place them in a sealable zip-lock container, and label them as hazardous drugs.
- Do not use IV containers designed with venting tubes, to prevent possible spillage.

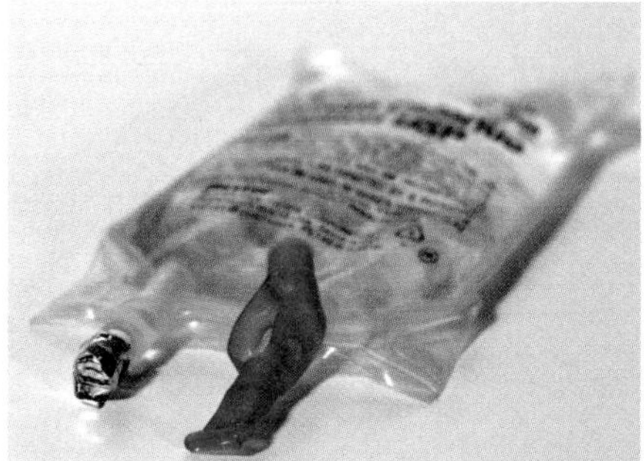

Figure 8-9 Covered IV ports

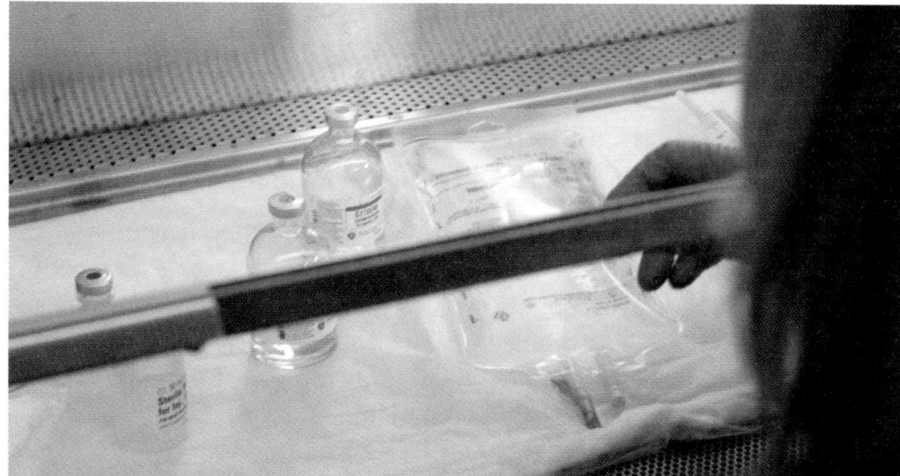

Figure 8-10 Final product

- Perform work with hazardous drugs in a BSC on a disposable, plastic-backed paper liner, which you should change after a spill or when sterile compounding is complete (Figure 8-10).

PHASEAL

Many pharmacy workplaces use a device known as the PhaSeal (Figures 8-11 and 8-12). This closed system, distributed by the Baxa Corporation, is designed to help reduce or eliminate human exposure to cancer chemotherapy drugs. The PhaSeal is a set of disposable containment devices used in drug mixing and administration that connect the original drug vial, the syringe, and the IV injection or infusion set together in a sealed pathway. It is constructed with a double membrane that prevents drug leakage; an expansion chamber equalizes the pressure in the system to prevent aerosols.

Use to attach PhaSeal injector to IV line for drug administration.

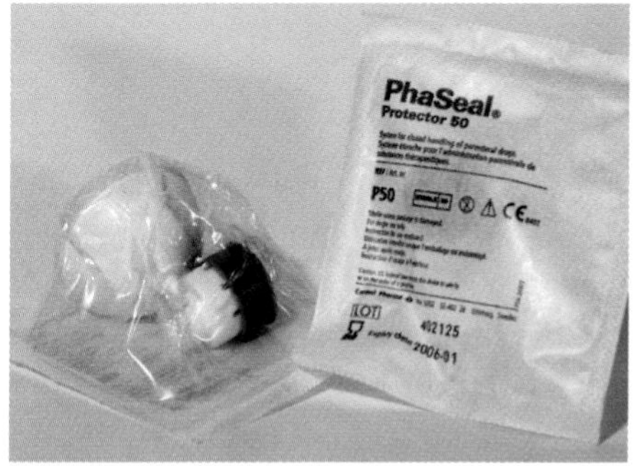

Figure 8-11 PhaSeal® Protector 50 - Protected needle for sealed transfer of fluids from vial to syringe and syringe to delivery device. Leur-lock connector.

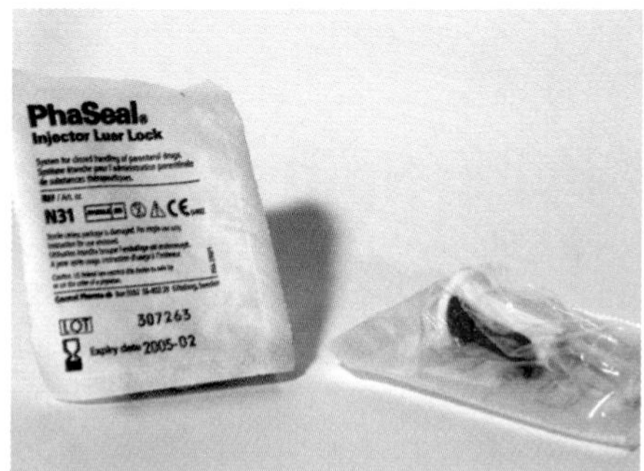

Figure 8-12 PhaSeal® Luer Lock Injector - Expansion chamber for standard-neck vials and 50-mL syringes or smaller. Holds up to 60 cc of air.

Disposal of Cytotoxic Medications

Dispose of all cytotoxic medications and related supplies in a yellow, puncture-resistant hazardous container identified as a chemotherapy waste container (Figure 8-13). There are no exceptions. This waste may include the following:

- Discarded gloves
- Disposable gowns
- Disposable goggles
- Any other disposable material used during chemotherapy administration, such as IV bags/bottles, tubing, and any unbreakable items

Typically, you will place these waste items in a sealed zip-lock bag before putting them in the waste container. Place needles and syringes in a standard puncture-proof sharps container without clipping or capping them.

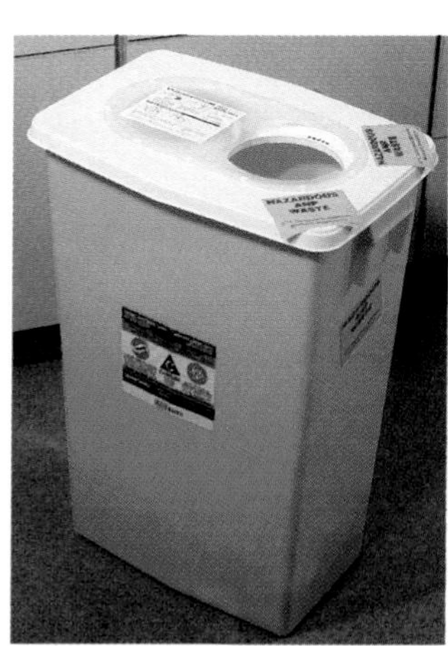

Figure 8-13 Chemotherapy waste container

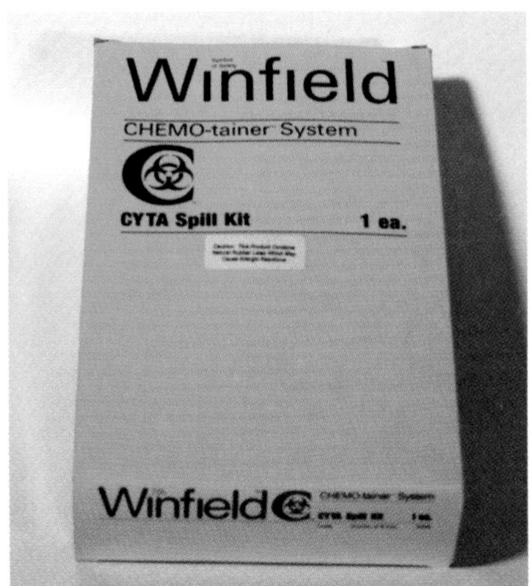

Figure 8-14 Chemo spill kit

Chemo Spills

Keep a chemo spill kit (Figure 8-14) available at all times nearby the mixing area. A chemo spill can occur when a person is in a hurry or not being careful. A chemo spill is never convenient, so be prepared.

As part of your orientation to chemotherapy compounding, take the time to read and reread information about chemo spill kits. Inevitably, chemo spills always occur during the most inappropriate times.

OSHA recommends that chemo spill kits be kept available at all times in areas that cytotoxic compounding occurs. The spill kit must be clearly labeled and contain the following items:

permeability the property or state of being penetrable

- Chemical splash goggles
- Low-**permeability** disposable gown and shoe covers or coveralls
- Two pairs of gloves (utility and latex gloves)
- Two sheets of absorbent, plastic-backed material
- 250-mL and 1-L spill control pillows
- Puncture-resistant sharps container
- Small scoop to collect glass fragments
- Two large, labeled, sealable hazardous drug waste disposal bags
- Appropriate respirator

There are two types of spills—large and small. The American Society of Health-System Pharmacists (ASHP) defines small spills as less than 5 mL or 5 g. Large spills are anything over 5 mL or 5 g.

OSHA suggests the following guidelines for cleaning small spills:

- Wipe up liquid spills with absorbent gauze pads.
- Wipe up solid spills with wet absorbent gauze.
- Clean spill areas three times using a detergent followed by clean water.

- Pick up broken glass fragments using a small scoop (never your hands) and place them in an appropriately labeled sharps container.

OSHA suggests the following guidelines for cleaning large spills:

- Gently cover liquid spills with absorbent sheets or spill-control pads or pillows.
- Clean up powder spills with damp cloths or towels.
- Use protective apparel, including respirators, if there is any suspicion of any airborne powder or aerosols.
- Thoroughly clean all contaminated surfaces three times with detergent and water. Avoid chemical inactivation in this setting.
- Place all contaminated absorbent sheets and other material in an appropriately labeled hazardous drug disposal bag.

ASHP Guidelines for Safe Handling of Cytotoxic Drugs

The ASHP Technical Assistance Bulletin on Handling Cytotoxic and Hazardous Drugs contains pertinent, valuable information. It is strongly advised that you become familiar with its content. This document provides several guidelines/suggestions from ASHP to help protect personnel and patients from accidental exposure, such as the following:

- Limit access.
- Identify and label all hazardous drugs.
- Educate the patient and family about any and all special precautions that might need to be taken.
- Have a written procedure in place for any chemo spills along with a chemo spill kit.
- Design facilities to prevent easy spillage and breakage (for example, place chemo drugs in a bin on a shelf rather than just on a shelf).
- Use a method for transportation designed to reduce spills, such as a cart with a rim.
- Maintain written policies and procedures for the preparation of chemotherapeutic agents.
- Conduct orientations for all employees to inform them about hazardous drugs.
- Implement yearly process validations to test the performance of the staff.
- Keep MSDS (Material Safety Data Sheets) for each individual hazardous drug easily accessible in the pharmacy.
- Engineer appropriate airflow and venting to protect the sterility of the product as well as to protect personnel from possible exposure.
- Require employees to wear appropriate apparel, including the following:
    - Gloves—disposable, surgical latex, and powder-free. ASHP recommends double-gloving (wearing two pairs of gloves).

    - Gown—disposable, lint-free, low-permeability fabric, with a solid front, long sleeves, and tight-fitting cuffs.
    - Respirator—must be worn if not working in a BSC.
    - Goggles—should be worn in situations where personnel may be exposed to potential eye contact.
- Design policies to outline proper aseptic technique.
- Train personnel in procedures for preparing and dispensing non-injectable hazardous drugs.
- Train personnel in procedures in case of accidental skin or eye exposure to hazardous drugs.
- Ensure that all hazardous drugs bear a CAUTION label.

A Final Caution

If you are pregnant, nursing, or thinking about becoming pregnant, avoid compounding cytotoxic agents—both IV and PO. Many hospitals have set guidelines for employees that fit into these categories. Remember that most cytotoxic (antineoplastic) drugs target fast-growing cells, including the ovaries and sperm. In addition, some chemotherapy drugs are mutagenic, which may increase the risk of miscarriages and birth defects.

The following are other risks associated with the handling of chemotherapy drugs:

- The drug may get out of the container and into the air.
- The drug may enter the handler's body through inhalation, absorption, ingestion, or accidental injection.
- The drug may cause cell damage.

Again, you can never be too careful when it comes to the safety and handling of these agents. Knowledge and practice are key.

CONCLUSION

Aseptic technique is necessary to protect both the patient and the preparer, especially in the case of cytotoxic or antineoplastic agents used in chemotherapy. These drugs are designed with one primary purpose: to kill or damage cells; they are non-discriminatory in the fact that they will damage the technician's cells just as easily as the targeted cells of the patient, if contact occurs. You must take special precautions when working with these agents; only experienced, trained, and validated technicians should be involved in the preparation of these products.

CHAPTER TERMS

aerosolization
suspension of small particles (liquid or powder) in the air

antineoplastic
a drug intended to inhibit or prevent the maturation and proliferation of neoplasms that may become malignant

biological safety cabinet (BSC)
a type of airflow hood in which chemotherapy drugs are compounded

carcinogenic
producing a malignant new growth that arises from the epithelium, which is found in skin or, more commonly, the lining of body organs

chemo mat
an absorbent mat used in the BSC over which the IV tech should compound cytotoxic agents so any spills can be absorbed

chemotherapy
treatment of cancer with drugs (chemicals)

cytotoxic
describes chemicals that are directly toxic to cells, preventing their reproduction or growth

malignant
tending to become progressively worse and to result in death

permeability
the property or state of being penetrable

shadowing
the act of blocking airflow in the BSC

teratogenic
tending to produce anomalies of formation

yellow hazardous disposal containers
containers used to dispose of hazardous medications and the equipment used to compound them; these containers require special disposal

CHAPTER REVIEW QUESTIONS

MULTIPLE CHOICE

1. What types of patients are diagnosed with cancer? __________.
   a. children
   b. women
   c. men
   d. geriatrics
   e. all of the above

2. What cells do chemotherapy agents target? __________.
   a. all cells
   b. slow-growing cells
   c. fast-growing cells
   d. carcinoma cells
   e. plasma cells

3. Which of the following are fast-growing cells? __________.
   a. tumors
   b. ovaries
   c. sperm
   d. T cells
   e. all of the above

4. When working in a biological safety cabinet (BSC), the IV technician must keep in mind the direction of the airflow to prevent shadowing. Where does shadowing occur in the BSC? __________.
   a. from the front of the hood
   b. from the back of the hood
   c. from the top of the hood
   d. from behind the operator
   e. shadowing does not occur in a BSC

5. All chemotherapy drugs and waste must be disposed of in a __________.
   a. yellow hazardous disposal container
   b. red biohazard container
   c. blue recycle bin
   d. oversized medical waste container
   e. stainless steel cart

6. What must be done to a pair of gloves before they enter the BSC? __________.
   a. They must be stretched out at least an inch.
   b. They must be prepowdered.
   c. They must be washed.
   d. They must be placed in the hood for 5 min.
   e. They must be placed to the left of the BSC.

7. Who is responsible for writing a chemotherapy order? __________.
   a. IV technician
   b. pharmacist
   c. nurse
   d. physician
   e. patient

8. Who is responsible for performing a final check on a chemotherapy medication? __________.
   a. IV technician
   b. pharmacist
   c. nurse
   d. physician
   e. patient

9. The HEPA filter must be recertified every __________ or if the hood is moved.
   a. two years
   b. evening
   c. six months
   d. year
   e. other day

10. Final products should be labeled and placed in __________.
   a. a sealable zip-lock container
   b. an airtight glass container
   c. an opaque container to protect from light
   d. a container with a carry handle
   e. a stainless steel container

11. A large spill is considered anything over _______.
   a. 1 oz.
   b. 10 mL
   c. 4 mL
   d. 5 mL

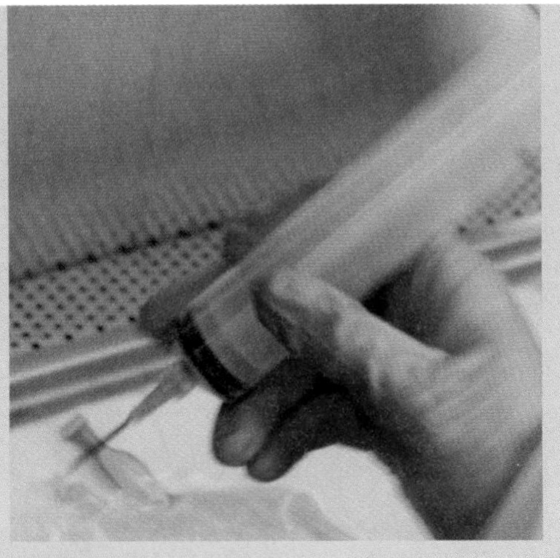

CHAPTER 9

Quality Control and Assurance

Learning Objectives

After completing this chapter, you should be able to:

- Explain the necessity of quality control.
- State tasks that require quality-assurance procedures.
- Help the pharmacist ensure the quality of all pharmaceutical services.
- List the principles of quality assurance to all pharmacy activities.
- Discuss the implications of USP Chapter 797.
- Compare the various risk levels for differing compounded sterile preparations and the quality-assurance requirements of each.

INTRODUCTION

Successful management of quality is not the sole responsibility of the quality manager nor the quality-assurance department. Each and every person involved in the pharmacy must understand the inherent responsibility that accompanies pharmaceuticals and their production. Quality-assurance activities are an absolute necessity in pharmacy. Each pharmacy aspect requires quality measurements to ensure integrity of the process and the final product. As someone who is involved in compounding sterile products, you must be completely aware of the potential consequences of poor quality control. Practicing proper aseptic technique is only one area subjected to quality-control measures.

Crucial to any product that is manufactured, including sterile compounds, and delivered to a patient population is a set of testing activities that determine the integrity of both the production process and the quality of the final product. Through careful design and validation of both the process and process controls, a manufacturer can establish a high degree of confidence that all manufactured units from successive lots will be acceptable. Pharmacy is a highly regulated arena and not without good reason. Sterile product preparation, if conducted poorly, has the potential for producing contaminated products that can harm patients and personnel. Problems due to cross-contamination, such as infection and even death, can result if strict procedures that limit the possibility of such exposure are not followed.

The importance of approved quality-control activities and measures cannot be emphasized enough in this text. Quality assurance should never be underestimated, nor any part of the process skipped for any reason. To do so would compromise public and patient safety.

Elements of Quality in Pharmacy

All pharmacy personnel must understand the basic rules of pharmacy when it comes to medication error prevention.

THE FIVE RIGHTS

The five rights are a simple checklist to be used at any point in the medication process. Ensuring that each item is correct allows very little room for error. The five rights are as follows:

- Right patient
- Right medication
- Right dose
- Right route of administration
- Right time

Know each one of these rights and do not forget them throughout your pharmacy career. Related criteria to the five rights are considerations such as the correct therapy for the patient's condition and stringent rules for the packaging and distribution of medications.

QUALITY-ASSURANCE FUNCTIONS

Numerous activities must be performed in order to ensure the integrity of the product and the production. These include written policies and procedures, documentation, personnel training, system checks and **process validation**, and daily assessment of all operations.

process validation
microbiological simulation of an aseptic process with growth medium processed in a manner similar to the processing of the product and with the same container or closure system

QUALITY IMPROVEMENT

In each facility subjected to quality-control measures, a process of quality improvement must also be in place. Quality improvement ensures that while processes are performed over time, integrity is not lost due to problems such as lack of training, equipment failure, outdated facilities, and other noncompliance issues. Essential to this process are activities such as monitoring trends, conducting audits, identifying and analyzing problems, taking corrective measures, conducting testing, and suggesting change. One particular area that has received a lot of attention is medication errors, which are usually the result of a system failure. Many facilities constantly revise their processes in an effort to minimize errors by closely evaluating each and every step involved. This is just one example of where quality-control measures are not only crucial to satisfy legal and other requirements, but crucial to public safety as well.

Guidelines

Various agencies issue guidelines to help establish standard practices and ensure universal testing procedures. Many regulatory agencies and professional associations have published guidelines for aseptic procedures and quality-control programs for pharmacy. These evolving standards cover both good manufacturing practices and quality-assurance programs.

FDA

The Food and Drug Administration (FDA) publishes Good Manufacturing Practices (GMP), which have been around for some time, and revises these guidelines as necessary. This set of standards offers guidelines for the compounding of sterile products, while another FDA document states guidelines on the manufacture of sterile products by aseptic processing. Included in these documents are quality system regulations, which will make standards consistent with quality system requirements.

JCAHO

The Joint Commission on Accreditation of Healthcare Organizations (JCAHO) publishes many general standards regarding pharmaceuticals and the facilities that manufacture, store, and deliver them. Like other organizations such as the FDA, JCAHO constantly revises its standards to improve compliance and keep up with the ever-evolving field of drugs and their manufacturing processes.

Through stringent inspections performed at timed intervals, JCAHO offers a highly respected and often necessary accreditation for health care organizations. JCAHO's focus is on the current state of health care and the potential for safer, higher-quality care. In addition to its published set of guidelines, JCAHO offers support to help organizations understand, participate, and comply with the accreditation process.

CDC

The Centers for Disease Control and Prevention (CDC) publish guidelines to assist in the prevention of spreading disease or infection. Since the primary goal of aseptic compounding mirrors these guidelines, it is easy to see why the CDC documents would be important to understand and put to practice.

CDC guidelines also provide invaluable information for hospital environment controls, especially where infection prevention is concerned.

ASHP

Some of the most widely recognized publications regarding quality assurance with sterile products, as well as all other pharmaceuticals and related information, are the guidelines established by the American Society of Health-System Pharmacists (ASHP). ASHP has taken an active role in producing documents addressing quality assurance. The ASHP *Guidelines on Quality Assurance for Pharmacy-Prepared Sterile Products* outlines the numerous considerations that are subjected to quality testing and assurance. It is a comprehensive document that addresses all areas impacted by quality assurance.

USP

The United States Pharmacopeia (USP) has published the first enforceable national standards for sterile compounding, USP Chapter 797. This major publication has gained the attention of numerous pharmacy regulatory entities, such as state boards of pharmacy, JCAHO, FDA, and many others. Agencies such as these are looking toward USP 797 as a universal guide, while amending and revising current publications.

MISCELLANEOUS

Other local, state, and national agencies also influence pharmacy practice and quality-assurance activities. They may also have recommended and established guidelines such as through state boards of pharmacy. Find out what rules apply in the state where you practice. It is extremely important that anyone who works in any area of pharmacy or related health care fields obtain copies of the preceding publications, read them, and understand their impact on the profession. Just as important is to reread these documents periodically, as edits, revisions, and amendments are suggested and made constantly.

WORKPLACE WISDOM

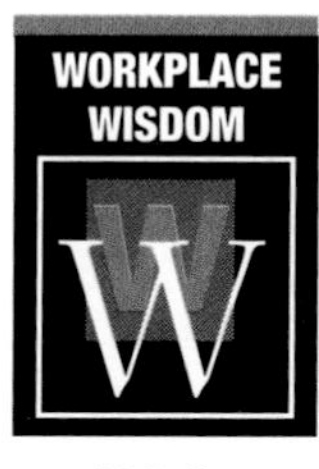

Room temperature refers to 15° to 30° C.
Refrigerated temperature is 2° to 8° C.
Freezer temperature is –20° to –10° C.

ASHP Guidelines on Quality Assurance for Pharmacy-Prepared Sterile Products

ASHP guidelines are divided into three risk levels and a discussion follows.

RISK LEVEL 1

Risk level 1 includes products that are stored at room temperature and completely administered within 28 hr of preparation; unpreserved, sterile, and prepared for administration to more than one patient and contain suitable preservatives; or prepared by a **closed-system aseptic transfer** of sterile, nonpyrogenic, finished pharmaceutical obtained from licensed manufacturers into sterile final containers obtained from licensed manufacturers.

closed-system aseptic transfer
the movement of sterile products from one container to another in which the containers, closure system, and transfer devices remain intact throughout the entire transfer process

Examples

Single patient admixtures; sterile ophthalmics; syringes without preservatives used within 28 hr; batch-prefilled syringes with preservatives; TPN solutions made by gravity transfer of carbohydrate and amino acid into an empty container with the addition of sterile additives with a needle and syringe.

Policies and Procedures (P&Ps)

compounding
the mixing of ingredients to prepare a medication for patient use

Up-to-date P&Ps for **compounding** sterile products should be available to all involved personnel. When policies are changed, they should be updated. Procedures should address personnel education, training, competency, product acquisition, storage, handling and delivery of final products, use and maintenance of facilities and equipment, garb and conduct of personnel, process validation, preparation technique, labeling, documentation, quality control, and material movement.

Personnel Training

All pharmacy personnel preparing sterile products should receive suitable didactic and experiential training and competency valuation through demonstration or testing (written or practical). In addition to the P&Ps listed previously, education includes chemical, pharmaceutical, and clinical properties of drugs and current good compounding practices.

Storage and Handling Inside the Pharmacy

Solutions, drugs, supplies, and equipment must be stored according to manufacturer or USP requirements. Refrigerator or freezer temperatures should be documented daily. Other storage areas should be inspected regularly to ensure that temperature, light, moisture, and ventilation meet requirements. Drugs and supplies should be shelved above the floor. Expired products must be removed from active product storage areas. Personnel traffic in storage areas should be minimized. Removal of products from boxes should be done outside **controlled areas**. Disposal of used supplies should be done at least daily. Product recall procedures must permit retrieving affected products from specific involved patients.

controlled area
the area designated for preparing sterile products; also called the clean room, in which the laminar airflow hood is located

Facilities and Equipment

Controlled areas should be separated from other operations to minimize unnecessary flow of materials and personnel through the area. Controlled areas must be clean, well lighted, and of sufficient size for sterile compounding. A sink with hot and cold water should be near, but not in, the controlled area. Controlled areas and inside equipment must be cleaned and disinfected regularly. Sterile products must be prepared in a class 200 environment (the critical areas) such as within a horizontal or vertical laminar airflow hood or barrier isolator. Computer entry, order processing, label generation, and record keeping should be performed outside the critical area.The critical area must be disinfected periodically. Airflow hoods should be recertified every six months or when moved, and prefilters should be changed periodically. Pumps should be recalibrated according to procedure.

Garb

In controlled areas, personnel must wear low-particulate, clean clothing covers such as clean gowns or coveralls with sleeves having elastic cuffs. Hand, finger, and wrist jewelry should be minimized or eliminated. Nails should be clean and trimmed. Gloves are recommended; those allergic to latex rubber must wear gloves made of a suitable alternative. Head and facial hair must be covered. Masks are recommended during aseptic preparation. Personnel preparing sterile products must scrub their hands and arms with an appropriate antimicrobial skin cleanser.

Aseptic Technique and Product Preparation

Sterile products must be prepared in a class 100 environment. Personnel must scrub their hands and forearms for an appropriate period at the beginning of each aseptic compounding process. Eating, drinking, and smoking are prohibited in the controlled area. Talking must be minimized to reduce airborne particles. Ingredients must be determined to be stable, compatible, and appropriate for the product to be prepared, according to manufacturer, USP, or scientific references. Ingredients must result in final products that meet physiological norms as to osmolality and pH for the intended route of administration. Ingredients and containers must be inspected for defects, expiration, and integrity before use. Only materials essential for aseptic compounding must be placed in the workbench. Surfaces of ampules and vials must be disinfected before placement in the workbench. Sterile components must be arranged in the workbench to allow uninterrupted laminar airflow over critical surfaces of needles, vials, ampules, and so on. Usually only one person and one preparation are allowed in the workbench at a time. Automated devices and equipment must be cleaned, disinfected, and placed in the workbench to enable laminar airflow. Aseptic technique must be used to avoid touch contamination of critical sites of containers and ingredients. Sterile powders must be completely reconstituted. Particles must be filtered from solutions. Needle cores must be avoided. The pharmacist must check before, during, and after preparation to verify the identity and amount of ingredients before release.

Process Validation

All personnel who prepare sterile products should pass a process validation of their aseptic technique before they prepare sterile products for patient use. Personnel competency should be reevaluated by process validation at least annually, whenever the quality-assurance program yields an unacceptable result, and whenever unacceptable techniques are observed. If microbial growth is detected, the entire sterile process must be evaluated, **corrective action** taken, and the process simulation test performed again.

corrective action
actions taken when the results of monitoring indicate a loss of control or when predetermined action levels are exceeded

Handling Sterile Products Outside the Pharmacy

Sterile products must be transported so as to be protected from excesses of temperatures and light. Transit time and condition should be specified. Delivery personnel should be trained as appropriate. Pharmacists must ascertain that the end user knows how to properly store products. End users must notify pharmacists when storage conditions are exceeded or when products expire so that pharmacists can arrange safe disposal or return.

Documentation

The following must be documented according to policy, laws, and regulations: training and competency evaluation of employees; refrigerator and freezer temperature logs; certification of workbenches; and other facility quality control logs as appropriate. Pharmacists must maintain appropriate records for the compounding and dispensing of sterile products.

Expiration Dating

All sterile products must bear an appropriate expiration date. Expiration dates should be assigned based on current drug stability information and sterility considerations. The pharmacist should consider all aspects of the final product, including drug reservoir, drug concentration, and storage conditions.

Labeling

Sterile products should be labeled with at least the following information: for patient-specific products, the patient's name and other appropriate patient identification; for batch-prepared products, control or lot numbers; all solution and ingredient names, amounts, strengths, and concentrations; expiration date (and time when applicable); prescribed administration regimen; appropriate auxiliary labeling; storage requirements; identification of the responsible pharmacist; any device-specific instructions; and any additional information, in accordance with state and federal regulations. A reference number for the prescription or order may also be helpful. The label should be legible and affixed to the product so that it can be read while being administered.

End-product Evaluations

The final product must be inspected for container leaks, integrity, solution cloudiness or phase separation, particulates in solution, appropriate solution color, and solution volume. The pharmacist must verify that the product was compounded accurately as to ingredients, quantities, containers, and reservoirs.

RISK LEVEL 2

Risk level 2 includes products that are administered beyond 28 hr after preparation and storage at room temperature; batch-prepared without preservatives and intended for use by more than one patient; or compounded by complex or numerous manipulations of sterile ingredients obtained from licensed manufacturers by using a closed-system aseptic transfer.

Examples

Injections for use in a portable pump or reservoir over multiple days; batch-reconstituted antibiotics without preservatives; batch-prefilled syringes without preservatives; TPN solutions mixed with an automatic compounding device.

Policies and Procedures

In addition to risk level 1 guidelines, procedures describe environmental monitoring devices and techniques, cleaning materials and disinfectants, equipment accuracy monitoring, limits of acceptability and corrective actions for environmental monitoring and process validation, master formula sheets and worksheets, personnel garb, lot numbers, and other quality-control methods.

Personnel Training

In addition to guidelines in risk level 1, training includes assessment of competency in all types of risk level 2 procedures via process simulation. Personnel must show competency in end product testing.

Storage and Handling Inside the Pharmacy

All guidelines for risk level 1 apply.

Facilities and Equipment

In addition to risk level 1 guidelines, controlled areas must meet class 10,000 clean room standards. Cleaning supplies should be selected to meet **clean room** standards. The **critical area** work surface must be cleaned between batches. Floors should be disinfected daily, equipment surfaces weekly, and walls monthly. There should be environmental monitoring of air and surfaces. An anteroom of high cleanliness is desirable. Automated compounding devices must be calibrated and verified as to accuracy according to procedure.

clean room
a room in which the concentration of airborne particles is controlled and where aseptic compounding takes place

critical area
any area in the controlled area where products and other materials are exposed to the environment

Garb

In addition to risk level 1 guidelines, gloves, gowns, and masks are required. During sterile preparation, gloves should be rinsed frequently with a suitable agent (such as 70% isopropyl alcohol) and changed when their integrity is compromised. Shoe covers are helpful in maintaining the cleanliness of the controlled area.

Aseptic Technique and Product Preparation

In addition to risk level 1 guidelines, a master worksheet containing formula, components, procedures, sample label, final evaluation, and testing is made for each product batch. A separate worksheet and lot number are used for each batch. When combining multiple sterile ingredients, a second pharmacist should verify calculations. The pharmacist should verify data entered into an automatic compounder before processing and check the end product for accuracy.

Process Validation

All risk level 1 guidelines apply, and process simulation procedures should cover all types of manipulations, products, and batch sizes that are encountered in risk level 2.

Handling Sterile Products Outside the Pharmacy

All guidelines for risk level 1 apply.

Documentation

In addition to the guidelines in risk level 1, documentation of end product testing and batch preparation records must be maintained according to policies, laws, and regulations.

Expiration Dating

All guidelines for risk level 1 apply.

Labeling

All guidelines for risk level 1 apply.

End-product Evaluations

In addition to risk level 1 guidelines, toxic products, such as concentrated glucose and potassium chloride, should be tested for accuracy of concentration.

RISK LEVEL 3

Risk level 3 includes products that are compounded from nonsterile ingredients or components, containers, or equipment before terminal sterilization; or prepared by combining multiple ingredients, sterile or nonsterile, by using an open-system transfer before terminal sterilization.

Examples

Alum bladder irrigation; morphine injection made from powder or tablets; TPN solutions made from dry amino acids or sterilized by final filtration; autoclaved IV solutions.

Policies and Procedures

Procedures cover every aspect of preparation of risk level 3 sterile products, so that all products have the identity, strength, quality, and purity purported for the product. Thirteen general P&Ps in addition to those in risk levels 1 and 2 are required.

Personnel Training

Operators must have specific education, training, and experience to prepare risk level 3 products. They must understand principles of good compounding practice for risk level 3 products including aseptic processing;

component and end product testing; sterilization; and selection and use of containers, equipment, and closures.

Storage and Handling Inside the Pharmacy

In addition to risk level 1 guidelines, procedures include procurement, identification, storage, handling, testing, and recall of components and finished products. Finished but untested products must be quarantined under a minimal risk for contamination or loss of identity in an identified quarantine area.

Facilities and Equipment

Products must be prepared in a class 100 workbench in a class 10,000 clean room, in a class 100 clean room, or in a suitable barrier isolator. Access to the clean room must be limited to those preparing the products who are in appropriate garb.

Methods are needed for cleaning, preparing, sterilizing, calibrating, and documenting the use of all equipment. Walls and ceilings should be disinfected weekly. All nonsterile equipment that is to come in contact with the sterilized final product should be sterilized before introduction into the clean room. An anteroom of high cleanliness (class 100,000) should be provided. Appropriate cleaning and disinfection of the environment and equipment are required.

Garb

In addition to risk level 1 and 2 guidelines, clean room garb must be worn inside the controlled area at all times during the preparation of risk level 3 sterile products. Attire consists of a low-shedding coverall, head cover, face mask, and shoe covers. Before donning this garb, personnel must thoroughly wash their hands and arms. Upon return to the controlled area or support area during processing, personnel should regown with clean garb.

Aseptic Technique and Product Preparation

In addition to risk level 1 and 2 guidelines, nonsterile components must meet USP standards for identity, purity, and endotoxin levels, as verified by a pharmacist. Batch master worksheets should also include comparisons of actual with anticipated yields, sterilization methods, and quarantine specifications.

Presterilized containers should be used if feasible. Final containers must be sterile and capable of maintaining product integrity throughout shelf life. Sterilization method is based on properties of the product. Final filtration methods require attention to many elements of product, filter, and filter integrity.

Process Validation

In addition to risk level 1 and 2 guidelines, written policies should be established to validate all processes (including all procedures, components, equipment, and techniques) for each risk level 3 product.

Handling Sterile Products Outside the Pharmacy

All guidelines for risk level 1 apply.

Documentation

In addition to risk level 1 and 2 guidelines, documentation for risk level 3 products must include a preparation worksheet, sterilization records if applicable, quarantine records if applicable, and end product evaluation and testing records.

Expiration Dating

In addition to risk level 1 and 2 guidelines, there must be a reliable method for establishing all expiration dates, including laboratory testing of product stability, pyrogenicity, and chemical content when necessary.

Labeling

All guidelines for risk level 1 and 2 apply.

End-product Evaluations

In addition to risk level 1 and 2 guidelines, the medium fill procedure should be supplemented with a program of end product sterility testing according to a formal sampling plan. Samples should be statistically adequate to reasonably ensure that batches are sterile. A method for recalling batch products should be established if end product testing yields unacceptable results. Each sterile preparation or batch must be laboratory tested for conformity to written specifications (such as for concentration and pyrogenicity). It is advisable to quarantine sterile products compounded from nonsterile components pending the results of end product testing.

Core Concepts from USP 797 and ASHP Guidelines

As previously mentioned, USP Chapter 797 is the first enforceable set of standards that define the responsibilities of many areas subjected to quality control. The ASHP guidelines and USP Chapter 797 publications offer a virtually unquestionable view as to what is necessary for the quality-control process. These publications are extremely complex and cannot possibly be covered fully in this one chapter; this is why it is important for you to read them yourself and understand their impact on your pharmacy career. Next, we will briefly describe some of the common considerations in these documents.

RISK LEVELS

Sterile products are grouped into three levels of risk depending on the potential risk of product integrity and patient safety. Risk level 1 includes products with the least potential risk, while risk level 3 includes those with the greatest. Risk levels define where a particular prepared product might be grouped. Each risk level has variant recommendations and guidelines as well, which aid in reducing contamination of all sorts.

Sometimes it can be confusing to decide under which risk level a specific product falls. A list of examples is provided to help clarify this so that you can understand all the guidelines that apply. In any case, it is always acceptable to follow the most stringent guidelines. As the saying goes, better safe than sorry!

POLICIES AND PROCEDURES

There is not a pharmacy in the United States that can operate without policies and procedures, which address updating, accessibility to personnel, accuracy, standard operating procedures (SOP), monitoring, and so much more. Not only do they apply to drug processes, but every single of aspect of pharmacy must have P&Ps. Every person working in a pharmacy has the responsibility of knowing the policies and procedures that impact them in their daily routines. Workplaces carry the responsibility of providing the P&Ps and keeping them updated. Know your policies and procedures.

PERSONNEL, EDUCATION, AND EVALUATION

We all know that it is important for personnel to have proper training and skills to perform their duties in pharmacy. Because pharmacy is ever-evolving, including areas of sterile products, personnel must also constantly update their skills and continue their education to stay abreast of this wealth of information. Facilities must have a process of evaluating the skills (assessment) and knowledge of their personnel to ensure that they are competent in their practice. Well-educated and well-trained professionals are key to minimizing risks and errors. This is a never-ending process that continues throughout your pharmacy career.

STORAGE AND HANDLING INSIDE AND OUTSIDE THE PHARMACY

Extremely important is how medications are packaged, prepared, and delivered. Once a final product is presented, it can easily be compromised if it is not stored or handled properly. For example, suppose that an IV solution that needs to be refrigerated is not placed in a refrigerator. Contamination ensues and the product is no longer safe to use. In addition to the waste that occurs, how can we ensure that the product does not reach the patient? The same can be said of preparation that is not done properly in an aseptic manner. Before the final product is delivered to the patient, it has already been compromised and could do great harm if the error goes undetected.

FACILITIES AND EQUIPMENT

Great care should be taken when designing a facility that will be performing aseptic compounding. All areas where actual compounding take place, in particular, are held to extremely high standards. As you have read in previous chapters, anterooms, critical areas, clean rooms, and many other areas fall under this category. In addition, all equipment and supplies used in aseptic compounding facilities must be installed properly, used properly, maintained, and monitored.

ASEPTIC TECHNIQUE, PRODUCT PREPARATION, AND GARB

Much emphasis is placed on the actual processes that take place during manufacturing. Any process that requires constant evaluation and improvement has many checkpoints. Major focus in this area is in the prevention of microbial contamination. All things considered here involve ingredients, components, proper gowning, and all supplies used in aseptic compounding.

PROCESS VALIDATION

The FDA defines process validation as "*establishing documented evidence which provides a high degree of assurance that a specific process will consistently produce a product meeting its pre-determined specifications and quality characteristics.*" Each stage in the validation of the overall process should proceed in accordance with a pre-established and formally approved, detailed, written protocol or series of related protocols. Personnel should be assessed as to their competency in performing and understanding these protocols. In addition, controls should be in place to prevent unauthorized changes to the processes or protocols, especially in the absence of relevant data. There are numerous requirements to the process validations themselves, such as identification numbers and specific methodology on how to obtain and test samples. Nothing is exempt from a process validation, including hand washing, aseptic technique, storage, and training. Even re-evaluating the validation process itself is subject to this control measure. Also included here are guidelines for corrective measures when integrity falters. A procedure must be in place to correct situations—everything from discovery, reporting, data collection, and corrective actions.

END-PRODUCT EVALUATION

After all the other considerations that have been addressed, now it is time for the final check. This is known as the end product evaluation. Pharmacy technicians may think this is the pharmacist's final check, but that is only a small part. Also included are inspections, more specifically with periodic sampling of batches manufactured under the exact same conditions and then tested.

Documentation and Labeling

Without a doubt, pharmacy requires extensive documentation of all sorts. All products dispensed must be labeled. All components used must be labeled. Every piece of equipment must have records. A pharmacy may have several methods or forms for different documentation needs. For example, standard operating procedures (SOPs) are records/documentation that illustrate how a product is made or processed. Having an SOP for each procedure not only ensures that each person about to prepare a product knows the correct procedure, but also ensures consistency with each preparation. A crucial part of any IV or chemotherapy preparation is documentation. Documentation is a record of patient information, product preparation, label information, and any other important information regarding the product or how it was made. For each product made for each patient, there must be documentation that includes information about the patient such as patient diagnosis, IV regimen, dosages, body surface area (BSA), lab values, and other pertinent information. Another part of this record is a worksheet that has information regarding the preparation and final product, such as ingredients, preparation or process, labeling, storage and handling information, expiration date, batch/lot identifying numbers, warnings, and other miscellaneous information.

Controlled substances require even more documentation than noncontrolled substances. Accurate and proper record keeping and documentation are essential and require strict guidelines to assure the origin of all components, the process performed, and all other things mentioned in this chapter.

Each facility may have its own forms, but the fundamentals are the same. Final products and processes have certain information such as that described previously, which must be included and kept for a time period to be determined based on the information, laws and regulations, and facility policy.

It is highly important that you become familiar with and understand how to fill out required documentation forms completely and accurately. This is an area of pharmacy that must not be overlooked at any time for any reason.

CONCLUSION

As previously stated, this chapter should not serve as a complete understanding of quality assurance and medications. The subject is complex and requires acute awareness of every aspect of pharmaceuticals and constant research to stay abreast. Each step of the manufacturing process must be controlled to ensure that the finished product meets all quality and design specifications. If you understand **quality-control** measures, however, you truly understand the necessity of everything you do. To recap, **quality assurance** involves the following:

- personnel training and competency
- various quality assurance steps
- environmental control and monitoring
- quality testing of compounded dosage forms
- personnel aseptic technique evaluation
- determination of product risk
- storage and beyond-use dating
- standard operating procedures

quality control
the set of testing activities used to determine that the ingredients, components (such as containers), and final sterile products prepared meet predetermined requirements for identity, purity, nonpyrogenicity, and sterility

quality assurance
the set of activities used to ensure that the processes used in the preparation of sterile drug products lead to products that meet predetermined standards of quality

Many publications offer guidelines to follow in order to prevent contamination and maintain and improve safety for the patient. USP 797 expands on many previously written documents and helps clarify specific measures pharmacies must take to sustain a national standard consistent with all practices.

CHAPTER TERMS

clean room
a room in which the concentration of airborne particles is controlled and where aseptic compounding takes place

closed-system aseptic transfer
the movement of sterile products from one container to another in which the containers, closure system, and transfer devices remain intact throughout the entire transfer process

compounding
the mixing of ingredients to prepare a medication for patient use

controlled area
the area designated for preparing sterile products; also called the clean room, in which the laminar airflow hood is located

corrective action
actions taken when the results of monitoring indicate a loss of control or when predetermined action levels are exceeded

critical area
any area in the controlled area where products and other materials are exposed to the environment

process validation
microbiological simulation of an aseptic process with growth medium processed in a manner similar to the processing of the product and with the same container or closure system

quality assurance
the set of activities used to ensure that the processes used in the preparation of sterile drug products lead to products that meet predetermined standards of quality

quality control
the set of testing activities used to determine that the ingredients, components (such as containers), and final sterile products prepared meet predetermined requirements for purity, nonpyrogenicity, and sterility

CHAPTER REVIEW QUESTIONS

MULTIPLE CHOICE

1. Right medication, dose, route, time and patient are referred to as __________.
   a. the patient bill of rights
   b. the five rights
   c. right medication administration
   d. right place, right time
   e. distribution rights

2. Compromising a quality-control measure may result in what devastating effect? __________
   a. termination from a job
   b. a change in the uniforms that are worn
   c. microbial contamination
   d. bad documentation
   e. changed expiration dates

3. __________ provides accreditation to facilities that have passed strict guidelines relating to patient care.
   a. Food and Drug Administration
   b. Drug Enforcement Agency
   c. United States Pharmacopeia
   d. Joint Commission on Accreditation of Healthcare Organizations
   e. HIPAA

4. __________ were the first enforceable national published standards regarding sterile products.
   a. HIPAA 797
   b. USP 297
   c. JCAHO 123
   d. CDC 597
   e. USP 797

5. What three criteria are involved in ensuring quality for personnel performing aseptic compounding? __________
   a. dressing, hand washing, continuing education
   b. training, education, attendance
   c. needle manipulation, hood cleaning, competency
   d. competency, training, education
   e. experience, didactic training, ability

6. Sampling finished products and testing for integrity falls under which topic of quality assurance? Choose the best answer. __________.
   a. process validation
   b. end product evaluation
   c. equipment and facilities
   d. labeling
   e. storage and handling

7. For aseptic technique and product preparation at risk level 1, a clean room must be class __________.
   a. 10,000
   b. 100
   c. 150
   d. 1000
   e. 1,000,000

8. Refrigerator temperatures for environmental control purposes refers to what range? __________
   a. 5° to 10° C
   b. 10° to 20° C
   c. 4° to 5° C
   d. 2° to 8° C
   e. 0° to 10° C

9. The __________ of equipment that will be used in sterile compounding must be validated before use.

   a. quality
   b. calibration
   c. documentation
   d. training
   e. type

10. What agency's publication will have the largest impact on future quality-control practices in pharmacy? __________

   a. United States Pharmacopeia
   b. NABP
   c. Food and Drug Administration
   d. Joint Commission on Accreditation of Healthcare Organizations
   e. Drug Enforcement Agency

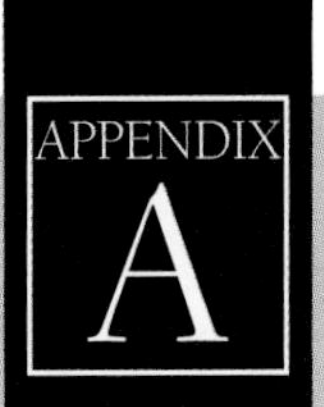

Terminology and Abbreviations

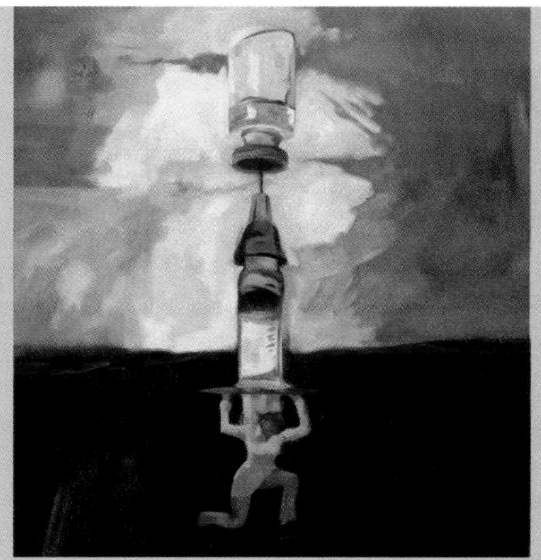

Terminology

acid describes a substance that increases the concentration of hydrogen ions (lowers the pH); an acidic substance is called an acid

additive a drug added to a solution intended for intravenous use

admixture a combination of two or more drug products for administration as one unit

aerosolization suspension of small particles (liquid or powder) in the air

albumin the protein of the highest concentration in plasma

alkaline describes a substance that decreases the concentration of hydrogen ions (raises the pH); an alkaline substance is called a base

amino acid any organic acid containing one or more amino groups ($-NH_2$) and one or more carboxyl groups ($-COOH$); amino acids are the building blocks of proteins

ampule sealed container, usually made of glass, containing a sterile medicinal solution, or a powder to be made up in solution, to be used for injection

anteroom the room located right outside the clean room, it is a low-particulate room, which means that it should not contain paper, boxes, or high-particulate matter. Food and drink should not be allowed in this room.

antibacterial an agent that destroys bacteria or inhibits their growth or reproduction

antibiotic a substance produced by a living organism capable of killing or inhibiting the growth of another microorganism (example: penicillin)

anticoagulant an agent that prevents or delays the clotting of blood (example: heparin)

antimicrobial an agent or action that kills or inhibits the growth of microorganisms

antineoplastic a drug intended to inhibit or prevent the maturation and proliferation of neoplasms that may become malignant

asepsis prevention of microbial contamination of living tissues or sterile materials by excluding, removing, or killing microorganisms

aseptic free from infection or septic material; sterile

aseptic technique the method used to manipulate sterile products so that they remain sterile

autoclave a steam sterilizer consisting of a metal chamber constructed to withstand the pressure that is required to raise the temperature of steam to the level required for sterilization

bacteriocidal an agent capable of killing bacteria

bacteriostatic capable of inhibiting the growth or reproduction of bacteria

barrel the part of a syringe that is marked with calibrations to designate the amount of liquid it contains

batch preparation the compounding of multiple sterile product units in a single process by the same individuals during one time period

bevel the tip of the needle, which is slanted to prevent coring when inserting it into a rubber diaphragm

biological safety cabinet (BSC) a type of hood in which chemotherapy drug are compounded

bolus an initial dose

buffer area the site where the laminar airflow hood is located

carcinogenic producing a malignant new growth that arises from the epithelium, which is found in skin or, more commonly, the lining of body organs

central line an IV access into one of the major blood vessels; this is the IV line through which hypertonic fluids may be given

chemo bags bags in which completed chemo IV bags or syringes are placed for transport; they can also be brought into the BSC for trash disposal to help minimize movement in and out of the BSC

chemo mat an absorbent mat placed in the BSC; the IV tech should compound cytotoxic agents on top of the chemo mat in case of any spills

chemo pin a pin that is very similar to a dispensing pin; however, the vented area of a chemo pin has a special filter to reduce any aerosolization of chemotherapy product

chemotherapy treatment of cancer with drugs (chemicals)

class 100 area contains no more than 100 particles 0.5 micron or larger for each cubic foot of air

clean room a room in which the concentration of airborne particles is controlled and where aseptic compounding takes place

closed-system transfer the movement of sterile products from one container to another in which the containers, closure system, and transfer devices remain intact throughout the entire transfer process

compatibility a feature of two or more components that can be mixed with each other without any physical and/or chemical stability problems in the admixture

compounding the mixing of ingredients to prepare a medication for patient use

contamination the act of introducing a harmful substance

controlled area the area designated for preparing sterile products; also called the clean room, in which the laminar airflow hood is located

coring transferring a part of the rubber stopper of a vial or container into a solution bag because of improper needle stick
corrective action actions taken when the results of monitoring indicate a loss of control or when predetermined action levels are exceeded
critical site any opening or pathway between the environment and the sterile product
cytotoxic describes chemicals that are directly toxic to cells, preventing their reproduction or growth
decompensate to fail to maintain adequate flow or amounts
desiccation the act of dehydrating or removing water content
diluent a liquid added to a solution to reduce its concentration
disinfectant an agent that is intended to kill or remove pathogenic microorganisms
electrolytes primary elements necessary for the proper function of the tissues of the human body (examples: potassium, sodium, magnesium)
enteral a method of nutrient delivery in which medication is given directly into the gastrointestinal tract
enzymes complex proteins that cause a specific chemical change in other substances without being changed themselves
epidural (EP) the route of administration whereby a drug is injected into the space surrounding the spinal cord
germicidal describes an agent that kills pathogenic microorganisms
gravity filling the free flow, due to gravity, of liquid from a container placed on a higher level to another one placed below
HEPA filter (high-efficiency particulate air) a filter capable of retaining 99.97 percent of all particles 0.3 micron or larger in diameter
heparin sulphated mucopolysaccharide, found in granules of mast cells, that inhibits the action of thrombin on fibrinogen by potentiating antithrombins, thereby interfering with the blood clotting cascade. Platelet factor IV will neutralize heparin
hub the bottom part of the needle, which is used to attach the needle to the syringe; it must remain sterile
hyperglycemia too high a level of glucose
hypertonic describes a solution with a greater concentration of dissolved substances than that of body fluids or blood cells; a solution with a concentration greater than 0.9% saline or greater than 5% dextrose; any solution with a greater osmotic pressure than that of human blood serum
hypoglycemia too low a level of glucose
hypotonic describes a solution with a lesser concentration of dissolved substances than that of body fluids or blood cells; a solution with a concentration less than 0.9% saline or less than 5% dextrose; any solution with a lesser osmotic pressure than that of human blood serum.
immunocompromised a condition in which the immune system is not functioning normally
infusion slow injection of a fluid into a vein
intramuscular (IM) the route of administration whereby a drug is injected into the muscle

intrathecal (IT) the route of administration whereby a drug is injected into the space surrounding the brain and spinal cord

intravenous (IV) the route of administration whereby a drug is injected into a vein

intravenous piggyback (IVPB) a small-volume IV fluid that normally has medication added

irrigation a solution used for washing

iso-osmotic having the same osmotic pressure

isotonic describes a solution in which body cells can be bathed without net flow of water across the semipermeable cell membrane; also describes a solution with the same tonicity as another solution

laminar airflow hood a specialized apparatus for preparing sterile pharmaceuticals, contains a special HEPA filter designed to provide a pathogen- and pyrogen-free workspace

loading dose an initial dose of a drug that is used to achieve a desired drug level

lyophilized describes a medication that comes in the form of a freeze-dried powder; it must be reconstituted before use

malignant tending to become progressively worse and to result in death

metathesis a mere change in place of a morbid substance, without removal from the body

narcotic a drug that is potentially addicting; sometimes used to relieve pain; a controlled substance

negative pressure occurs when the pressure outside a vial or bottle is greater than the pressure inside it, creating a partial vacuum; use negative pressure when working with ceftazidime, chemotherapy drugs, Mannitol, and any other drugs as instructed, as too much pressure will cause these drugs to leak from the vial

neonate a newborn baby

osmolality the concentration of solute in a solution per unit of solvent; commonly expressed as milliosmoles per kilogram

osmolarity the concentration of solute in a solution per unit of solution; commonly expressed as milliosmoles per liter

osmosis the tendency of a solvent to pass through a semipermeable membrane (such as the cell wall) into a solution of higher concentration to equalize concentrations on both sides of the membrane

parenteral administration via injection

particulates small matter

pathogen any disease-causing organism

peripheral line an IV line administered through a peripheral vein (usually in the arm or leg); any IV that is not through a central line. It is critical that only hypotonic solutions be administered through peripheral IV lines because hypertonic solutions can damage the vein

permeability the property or state of being penetrable

phlebitis inflammation of a vein

piggyback (IVPB) delivery of a secondary IV solution from an outside source into an IV line containing fluid from an existing line

positive pressure occurs when the pressure inside a vial or bottle is greater than the pressure outside it. It is sometimes helpful to use positive pressure when drawing up large volumes of solutions; the plunger will drift back by a volume equal to the amount of air added, thereby requiring less energy to withdraw fluid

preservative any additive intended to extend the content, stability, or sterility of active ingredients

process validation microbiological simulation of an aseptic process with growth medium processed in a manner similar to the processing of the product and with the same container or closure system

protocol the standard plan for a course of medical treatment

pyrogen a substance that produces fever

quality assurance the set of activities used to ensure that the processes used in the preparation of sterile drug products lead to products that meet predetermined standards of quality

quality control the set of testing activities used to determine that the ingredients, components (such as containers), and final sterile products prepared meet predetermined requirements for identity, purity, nonpyrogenicity, and sterility

reconstitute to add a diluent to a vial to create a liquid

renal failure loss of the kidneys' ability to excrete wastes, concentrate urine, and conserve electrolytes

sanitization a process that reduces microbial contamination to a low level by the use of cleaning solutions, hot water, or chemical disinfectants

sepsis the presence of organisms in the blood

shadowing the act of blocking airflow in the BSC

single dose vial (SDV) a vial that contains no preservatives; once the container is entered, contaminants may have been introduced and the container is no longer sterile

solute any substance that dissolves another substance

specific gravity the weight of a substance compared (as a ratio) with that of an equal volume of water

sterility the state of being free from microorganisms

sticky mats mats placed on the floor in the entrance from the anteroom to the clean room. The mats have multiple layers of sticky sheets that can be removed one layer at a time. The mats remove any particulates that may be carried into the clean room on the bottoms of the feet

subcutaneous (SC, SQ) the route of administration whereby a drug is injected beneath the skin

teratogenic tending to produce anomalies of formation

vial a small bottle or container that holds products such as injectable medications

yellow hazardous disposal containers containers used to dispose of hazardous medications and the equipment used to compound them; these containers require special disposal

Abbreviations

ACPE American College of Pharmaceutical Education
AHF Antihemolytic factor (Factor VIII, Factor IX)
amp ampule
ASHP American Society of Health-System Pharmacists
BSC biological safety cabinet
epi epinephrine
gtt. drops
ID intradermal
IgG immune globulin
IM intramuscular
inj injection
IT intrathecal
IV intravenous
IVP IV push
IVPB intravenous piggyback
KVO keep veins open
LAH laminar airflow hood
LVP large-volume parenteral
mag bags magnesium sulfate bags used in L&D (labor and delivery)
MDV multidose vials
MVI multivitamin injectable or PO (by mouth)
NPO nothing by mouth
NTG nitroglycerin
PCA personal controlled anesthesia
PCN penicillin
PF preservative-free
PRN as needed
qs a sufficient quantity of fluid added to a solution to raise it to the desired volume
SAS sterile antibiotic solution
SDV single dose vial
SW sterile water
SWFI sterile water for injection
TCN tetracycline
TKO to keep open; a rate fast enough to keep the vein open
TPA tissue plasminogen activator
vit. B_1 thiamine
vit. B_6 pyridoxine
vit. B_{12} cyanocobalamin
vit. C ascorbic acid
vit. K phytonadione, mephyton

Chemical Abbreviations

Ca calcium
Cl chloride
Cu copper

K potassium
K^+ potassium ion
KCl potassium chloride
K_3PO_4 potassium phosphate
Mg magnesium
$MgSO_4$ magnesium sulfate
MS or MSO_4 morphine sulfate
Na sodium
Na^+ sodium ion
NaCl sodium chloride
$NaHCO_3$ sodium bicarbonate
$NaPO_4$ sodium phosphate
PO_4 phosphate
SO_4 sulfate
Zn zinc

Measurement Abbreviations

gm gram
kg kilogram
mg milligram
mcg microgram
mEq milliequivalent
L liter
mL milliliter
U International Unit

IV Admixture Fluid Abbreviations

D70 dextrose 70% in water
D50 dextrose 50% in water
D10W dextrose 10% in water
D5W dextrose 5% in water
D5NS dextrose 5% in normal saline
D5$\frac{1}{2}$NS dextrose 5% in 0.45% normal saline
D5$\frac{1}{2}$NS w/20 mEq KCl dextrose 5% in 0.45% normal saline with 20 mEq of potassium chloride
D5$\frac{1}{4}$NS dextrose 5% in 0.225% normal saline
NS normal saline (0.9% sodium chloride)
$\frac{1}{2}$NS 0.45% normal saline
$\frac{1}{4}$NS 0.225% normal saline (0.2% on IV bags)
D5LR dextrose 5% in lactated Ringer's
LR lactated Ringer's

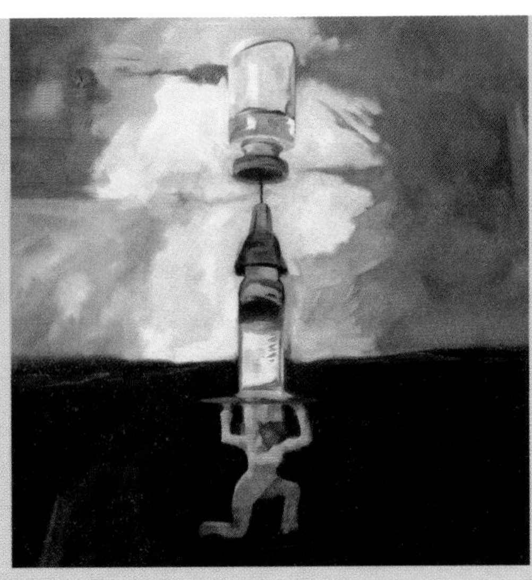

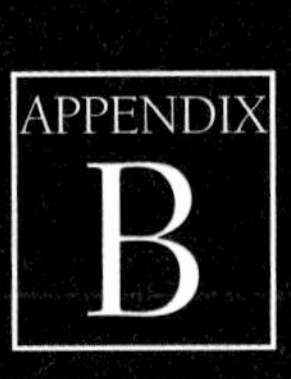

APPENDIX B

Common Intravenous Medications

Alphabetical—Generic Name

Generic Name	Brand Name	Use
acetazolamide Na	Diamox	antiglaucoma; anticonvulsant; diuretic; urinary alkalinizer
acyclovir	Zovirax	antiviral
aminophylline	Theophylline	bronchodilator; respiratory stimulant
aztreonam	Azactam	antibacterial
cefazolin Na	Ancef; Kefzol	antibacterial
cefoperazone Na	Cefobid	antibacterial
cefotaxime Na	Claforan	antibacterial
cefotetan	Cefotan	antibacterial
cefoxitin Na	Mefoxin	antibacterial
ceftazidime	Ceptaz; Fortaz	antibacterial
ceftizoxime Na	Cefizox	antibacterial
ceftriaxone Na	Rocephin	antibacterial
cefuroxime Na	Kefurox; Zinacef	antibacterial
cimetidine	Tagamet	antiulcer; gastric acid inhibitor
clindamycin	Cleocin	antibacterial; antiprotozoal
dexamethasone	Decadron	anti-inflammatory; antiemetic; immunosuppressant
dobutamine HCl	Dobutrex	inotropic agent; cardiac stimulant
dopamine HCl	Intropin	inotropic agent; cardiac stimulant; vasopressor
doxycycline	Vibramycin; Doxy	antibacterial; antiprotozoal; antimalarial
epinephrine HCl	Adrenalin Chloride	cardiac stimulant; bronchodilator; antiallergic; vasopressor
famotidine	Pepcid	antiulcer; gastric acid inhibitor
furosemide	Lasix	diuretic; antihypertensive; antihypercalcemic
gentamicin	Garamycin	antibacterial
heparin Na	Hep-Lock; Hep-Flush	anticoagulant
hydromorphone HCl	Dilaudid	narcotic analgesic
imipenem-cilastatin	Primaxin	antibacterial
isoproterenol	Isuprel	cardiac stimulant; bronchodilator; antiarrhythmic
kanamycin	Kantrex	antibacterial

Alphabetical—Generic Name

Generic Name	Brand Name	Use
labetalol	Normodyne; Trandate	alpha/beta-adrenergic blocking agent; antihypertensive
lidocaine	Xylocaine	antiarrhythmic
meperidine HCl	Demerol	narcotic analgesic; anesthesia adjunct
meropenem	Merrem	antibacterial
metoclopramide HCl	Reglan	GI stimulant; antiemetic
morphine	Astramorph; Duramorph	narcotic analgesic; anesthesia adjunct
nafcillin Na	Nafcil; Nallpen	antibacterial
nitroglycerin	Nitro-Bid; Tridil	antianginal; antihypertensive; vasodilator
norepinephrine	Levophed	vasopressor
ondansetron HCl	Zofran	antiemetic
oxacillin Na	Bactocill; Prostaphlin	antibacterial
pancuronium	Pavulon	neuromuscular blocking agent; anesthesia adjunct
pentobarbital Na	Nembutal Na	barbiturate; sedative; anticonvulsant
piperacillin/tazobactam	Zosyn	antibacterial
prochlorperazine	Compazine	antiemetic; antipsychotic
promethazine	Phenergan	antiemetic; sedative
propranolol	Inderal	beta-adrenergic blocking agent; antiarrhythmic
ranitidine	Zantac	H_2 antagonist; antiulcer agent; gastric acid inhibitor
succinylcholine	Anectine	neuromuscular blocking agent; anesthesia adjunct
thiopental	Pentothal Na	barbiturate; general anesthetic; anticonvulsant
thymoglobulin	Antithymocyte Globulin	immunosuppressant
tranexamic acid	Cyklokapron	antifibrinolytic; antihemorrhagic
warfarin	Coumadin	anticoagulant
zidovudine	Retrovir	antiviral

Alphabetical—Brand Name

Brand Name	Generic Name	Use
Adrenalin Chloride	epinephrine HCl	cardiac stimulant; bronchodilator; antiallergic; vasopressor
Ancef; Kefzol	cefazolin Na	antibacterial
Anectine	succinylcholine	neuromuscular blocking agent; anesthesia adjunct
Antithymocyte Globulin	thymoglobulin	immunosuppressant
Astramorph; Duramorph	morphine	narcotic analgesic; anesthesia adjunct
Azactam	aztreonam	antibacterial
Bactocill; Prostaphlin	oxacillin Na	antibacterial
Cefizox	ceftizoxime Na	antibacterial
Cefobid	cefoperazone Na	antibacterial
Cefotan	cefotetan	antibacterial
Ceptaz; Fortaz	ceftazidime	antibacterial
Claforan	cefotaxime Na	antibacterial
Cleocin	clindamycin	antibacterial; antiprotozoal
Compazine	prochlorperazine	antiemetic; antipsychotic
Coumadin	warfarin	anticoagulant
Cyklokapron	tranexamic acid	antifibrinolytic; antihemorrhagic
Decadron	dexamethasone	anti-inflammatory; antiemetic; immunosuppressant
Demerol	meperidine HCl	narcotic analgesic; anesthesia adjunct
Diamox	acetazolamide Na	antiglaucoma; anticonvulsant; diuretic; urinary alkalinizer
Dilaudid	hydromorphone HCl	narcotic analgesic
Dobutrex	dobutamine HCl	inotropic agent; cardiac stimulant

Alphabetical—Brand Name

Brand Name	Generic Name	Use
Garamycin	gentamicin	antibacterial
Hep-Lock; Hep-Flush	heparin Na	anticoagulant
Inderal	propranolol	beta-adrenergic blocking agent; antiarrhythmic
Intropin	dopamine HCl	inotropic agent; cardiac stimulant; vasopressor
Isuprel	isoproterenol	cardiac stimulant; bronchodilator; antiarrhythmic
Kantrex	kanamycin	antibacterial
Kefurox; Zinacef	cefuroxime Na	antibacterial
Lasix	furosemide	diuretic; antihypertensive; antihypercalcemic
Levophed	norepinephrine	vasopressor
Mefoxin	cefoxitin Na	antibacterial
Merrem	meropenem	antibacterial
Nafcil; Nallpen	nafcillin Na	antibacterial
Nembutal Na	pentobarbital Na	barbiturate; sedative; anticonvulsant
Nitro-Bid; Tridil	nitroglycerin	antianginal; antihypertensive; vasodilator
Normodyne; Trandate	labetalol	alpha/beta-adrenergic blocking agent; antihypertensive
Pavulon	pancuronium	neuromuscular blocking agent; anesthesia adjunct
Pentothal Na	thiopental	barbiturate; general anesthetic; anticonvulsant
Pepcid	famotidine	antiulcer; gastric acid inhibitor
Phenergan	promethazine	antiemetic; sedative
Primaxin	imipenem-cilastatin	antibacterial
Reglan	metoclopramide HCl	GI stimulant; antiemetic
Retrovir	zidovudine	antiviral
Rocephin	ceftriaxone Na	antibacterial
Tagamet	cimetidine	antiulcer; gastric acid inhibitor
Theophylline	aminophylline	bronchodilator; respiratory stimulant
Vibramycin; Doxy	doxycycline	antibacterial; antiprotozoal; antimalarial
Xylocaine	lidocaine	antiarrhythmic
Zantac	ranitidine	H_2 antagonist; antiulcer agent; gastric acid inhibitor
Zofran	ondansetron HCl	antiemetic
Zosyn	piperacillin/tazobactam	antibacterial
Zovirax	acyclovir	antiviral

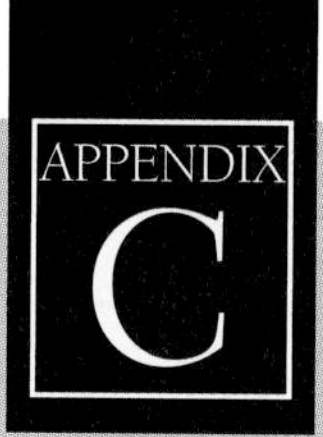

Training and Validation Forms

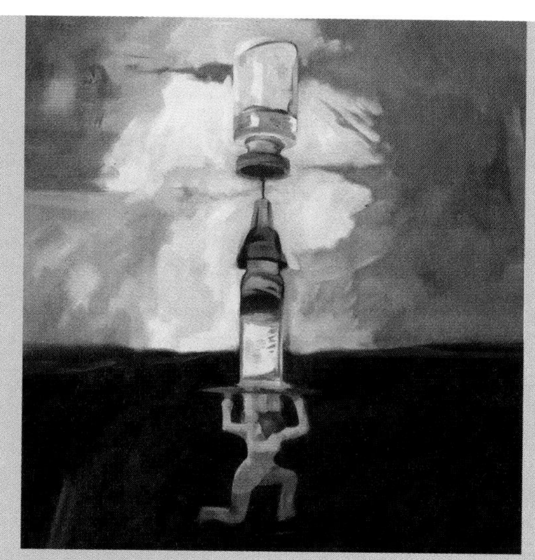

Figure C-1

Aseptic Technique Training Log

Student Name	
Date	
Start Time	
End Time	
Contact Hour(s)	
Location	
Trainer's Name	
Trainer's Lic. #	
State of License	
Daytime Phone (trainer)	
Skill(s) Covered	

By signing below, I validate that the information listed above is complete and fully accurate.

Student Signature Date Trainer Signature Date

Figure C-2

Aseptic Technique Training Log

Student Name	
Date	
Start Time	
End Time	
Contact Hour(s)	
Location	
Trainer's Name	
Trainer's Lic. #	
State of License	
Daytime Phone (trainer)	
Skill(s) Covered	

By signing below, I validate that the information listed above is complete and fully accurate.

Student Signature Date Trainer Signature Date

Figure C-3

Aseptic Technique Training Log

Student Name	
Date	
Start Time	
End Time	
Contact Hour(s)	
Location	
Trainer's Name	
Trainer's Lic. #	
State of License	
Daytime Phone (trainer)	
Skill(s) Covered	

By signing below, I validate that the information listed above is complete and fully accurate.

Student Signature	Date	Trainer Signature	Date

Aseptic Technique Training Log

Figure C-4

Student Name	
Date	
Start Time	
End Time	
Contact Hour(s)	
Location	
Trainer's Name	
Trainer's Lic. #	
State of License	
Daytime Phone (trainer)	
Skill(s) Covered	

By signing below, I validate that the information listed above is complete and fully accurate.

Student Signature Date

Trainer Signature Date

Figure C-5

Aseptic Technique Training Log

Student Name	
Date	
Start Time	
End Time	
Contact Hour(s)	
Location	
Trainer's Name	
Trainer's Lic. #	
State of License	
Daytime Phone (trainer)	
Skill(s) Covered	

By signing below, I validate that the information listed above is complete and fully accurate.

Student Signature	Date	Trainer Signature	Date

Aseptic Technique Training Log

Figure C-6

Student Name	
Date	
Start Time	
End Time	
Contact Hour(s)	
Location	
Trainer's Name	
Trainer's Lic. #	
State of License	
Daytime Phone (trainer)	
Skill(s) Covered	

By signing below, I validate that the information listed above is complete and fully accurate.

Student Signature Date

Trainer Signature Date

Figure C-7

Aseptic Technique Training Log

Student Name	
Date	
Start Time	
End Time	
Contact Hour(s)	
Location	
Trainer's Name	
Trainer's Lic. #	
State of License	
Daytime Phone (trainer)	
Skill(s) Covered	

By signing below, I validate that the information listed above is complete and fully accurate.

Student Signature　　Date　　Trainer Signature　　Date

Aseptic Technique Training Log

Figure C-8

Student Name	
Date	
Start Time	
End Time	
Contact Hour(s)	
Location	
Trainer's Name	
Trainer's Lic. #	
State of License	
Daytime Phone (trainer)	
Skill(s) Covered	

By signing below, I validate that the information listed above is complete and fully accurate.

Student Signature Date   Trainer Signature Date

Figure C-9

Aseptic Technique Training Log

Student Name	
Date	
Start Time	
End Time	
Contact Hour(s)	
Location	
Trainer's Name	
Trainer's Lic. #	
State of License	
Daytime Phone (trainer)	
Skill(s) Covered	

By signing below, I validate that the information listed above is complete and fully accurate.

Student Signature Date

Trainer Signature Date

Figure C-10

Aseptic Technique Training Log

Student Name	
Date	
Start Time	
End Time	
Contact Hour(s)	
Location	
Trainer's Name	
Trainer's Lic. #	
State of License	
Daytime Phone (trainer)	
Skill(s) Covered	

By signing below, I validate that the information listed above is complete and fully accurate.

Student Signature Date Trainer Signature Date

Figure C-11

Process Validation Record

Aseptic Hand Washing Technique

Student Name: ______________________________ Date: ____________

PROCEDURE	Yes	No
Removed all jewelry, watches, and objects up to the elbow		
Did not have on acrylic nails or nail polish		
Started water and adjusted to the appropriate temperature		
Avoided unnecessary splashing during process		
Used sufficient disinfecting agent/cleanser		
Cleaned all four surfaces of each finger		
Cleaned all surfaces of hands, wrists, and arms up to the elbows in a circular motion		
Did not touch the sink, faucet, or other objects that could contaminate hands		
Rinsed off all soap residue		
Rinsed hands, holding them upright and allowing water to drip to the elbow		
Did not turn off water until hands were completely dry		
Turned water off with a clean, dry, lint-free paper towel		
Did not touch the faucet while turning off the water		

By signing below, I certify that the student has demonstrated 100% competency at the above task.

____
Trainer Name (printed)

____
Trainer Signature

______________________________ ______________________________
Trainer Daytime Phone Trainer's License #

______________________________ ______________________________
Date State Licensed

Figure C-12

Process Validation Record

Horizonal Laminar Airflow Hood

Student Name: ______________________ Date: __________

PROCEDURE	Yes	No
Hood was turned on and running at least 30 min prior to preparation		
Followed proper hand-washing procedure and technique		
Wore appropriate apparel		
Used clean, sterile gauze/sponge and plenty of disinfectant to clean the hood		
Cleaned the IV pole first (if applicable)		
Cleaned the sides of the hood second, starting at the top and working side to side with overlapping strokes		
Cleaned the work surface last, starting at the back and working side to side with overlapping strokes		
Did not contaminate previously cleaned surfaces		
Did not block airflow from HEPA filter		
Did not utilize outer 6 in. of the hood opening		
Properly stood outside the hood without allowing the head to enter the inside		
Knew that hood certification is every six months, if moved, or if damaged		
Knew that prefilters should be changed monthly		

By signing below, I certify that the student has demonstrated 100% competency at the above task.

____
Trainer Name (printed)

____
Trainer Signature

____
Trainer Daytime Phone

____
Trainer's License #

____
Date

____
State Licensed

Figure C-13

Process Validation Record

Vertical Laminar Airflow Hood

Student Name: ______________________ Date: __________

PROCEDURE	Yes	No
Hood was turned on and running at least 30 min prior to preparation		
Followed proper hand-washing procedure and technique		
Wore appropriate apparel		
Used clean, sterile gauze/sponge and plenty of disinfectant to clean the hood		
Cleaned the IV pole first (if applicable)		
Cleaned the sides of the hood second, starting at the top and working side to side with overlapping strokes		
Cleaned the back wall and inside the glass shield, starting at the top and working up and down with overlapping strokes		
Cleaned the work surface last, starting at the back and working side to side with overlapping strokes		
Did not contaminate previously cleaned surfaces		
Did not lower the glass shield more than 8 in. from the work surface prior to preparation		
Did not block airflow from HEPA filter or air intake grills at any time		
Did not utilize outer 6 in. of the hood opening		

By signing below, I certify that the student has demonstrated 100% competency at the above task.

____
Trainer Name (printed)

____
Trainer Signature

____
Trainer Daytime Phone

____
Trainer's License #

____
Date

____
State Licensed

Figure C-14

Process Validation Record

Ampule Preparation

Student Name: ______________________ Date: ____________

PROCEDURE	Yes	No
Followed proper hand-washing procedure and technique		
Wore appropriate apparel		
Followed proper procedure and technique in cleaning the hood		
Performed all necessary calculations correctly prior to drug preparation		
Brought the correct drugs and concentrations into the hood for preparation		
Brought the correct supplies into the hood prior to preparation		
Inspected all products for particulate matter/contamination prior to use		
Cleared ampule neck of fluid before breaking		
Cleaned ampule neck correctly before breaking		
Wrapped ampule neck correctly before breaking		
Broke ampule correctly		
Attached filter device to syringe correctly		
Draw up ampule correctly, without spilling contents		
Removed filter needle and replaced it with new needle prior to injecting final container		
Drew up the correct amount of drug and checked measurement prior to injecting into container		
Cleaned additive port on final container prior to injecting drug		
Did not core or puncture side of additive port when adding drug to the final container		
Properly mixed contents of container and inspected for incompatibilities or particulate matter		
Properly sealed additive port of container		
Did not contaminate the needle or syringe during preparation		
Did not contaminate the hood		
Did not block airflow from HEPA filter or air intake grills at any time		
Did not utilize outer 6 in. of the hood opening		
Properly discarded all waste, including sharps		

By signing below, I certify that the student has demonstrated 100% competency at the above task.

____
Trainer Name (printed)

____
Trainer Signature

______________________ ______________________
Trainer Daytime Phone Trainer's License #

______________________ ______________________
Date State Licensed

Figure C-15

Process Validation Record

Ampule Preparation

Student Name: ______________________ Date: __________

PROCEDURE	Yes	No
Followed proper hand-washing procedure and technique		
Wore appropriate apparel		
Followed proper procedure and technique in cleaning the hood		
Performed all necessary calculations correctly prior to drug preparation		
Brought the correct drugs and concentrations into the hood for preparation		
Brought the correct supplies into the hood prior to preparation		
Inspected all products for particulate matter/contamination prior to use		
Cleared ampule neck of fluid before breaking		
Cleaned ampule neck correctly before breaking		
Wrapped ampule neck correctly before breaking		
Broke ampule correctly		
Attached filter device to syringe correctly		
Draw up ampule correctly, without spilling contents		
Removed filter needle and replaced it with new needle prior to injecting final container		
Drew up the correct amount of drug and checked measurement prior to injecting into container		
Cleaned additive port on final container prior to injecting drug		
Did not core or puncture side of additive port when adding drug to the final container		
Properly mixed contents of container and inspected for incompatibilities or particulate matter		
Properly sealed additive port of container		
Did not contaminate the needle or syringe during preparation		
Did not contaminate the hood		
Did not block airflow from HEPA filter or air intake grills at any time		
Did not utilize outer 6 in. of the hood opening		
Properly discarded all waste, including sharps		

By signing below, I certify that the student has demonstrated 100% competency at the above task.

____
Trainer Name (printed)

____
Trainer Signature

____
Trainer Daytime Phone

____
Trainer's License #

____
Date

____
State Licensed

Figure C-16

Process Validation Record

TPN Preparation

Student Name: ______________________ Date: __________

PROCEDURE	Yes	No
Followed proper hand-washing procedure and technique		
Wore appropriate apparel		
Followed proper procedure and technique in cleaning the hood		
Performed all necessary calculations correctly, prior to drug preparation		
Brought the correct drugs and concentrations into the hood for preparation		
Brought the correct supplies into the hood prior to preparation		
Inspected all products for particulate matter/contamination prior to use		
Withdrew electrolytes from vial according to proper procedures		
Added electrolytes to bottle of dextrose utilizing the vacuum inside the container		
Did not combine calcium- and phosphate-containing electrolytes inside the dextrose container		
Combined dextrose and amino acid solutions by adding to TPN bag		
Added phosphate-containing electrolytes to TPN bag after dextrose, amino acid, and other electrolytes had been added		
Visually inspected TPN for particulate contamination		
Added lipids last, if order called for a 3 in 1		
Properly mixed contents of TPN container		
Properly sealed additive port of TPN container		
Properly disconnected tubing from TPN bag and removed all air		
Properly sealed TPN bag where base solution was added		
Did not contaminate the needle or syringe during preparation		
Did not contaminate the hood		
Did not block airflow from HEPA filter or air intake grills at any time		
Did not utilize outer 6 in. of the hood opening		
Properly discarded all waste, including sharps		

By signing below, I certify that the student has demonstrated 100% competency at the above task.

______________________ ______________________

Trainer Name (printed) Trainer Signature

Figure C-17

Process Validation Record

Ampule Preparation—Hazardous Drugs

Student Name: ______________________________ Date: ____________

PROCEDURE	Yes	No
Followed proper hand-washing procedure and technique		
Wore appropriate apparel		
Followed proper procedure and technique in cleaning the hood		
Knew location of spill kit		
Knew location of eye wash station		
Performed all necessary calculations correctly prior to drug preparation		
Placed prep mat/paper drape correctly prior to drug preparation		
Brought the correct drugs and concentrations into the hood for preparation		
Brought the correct supplies into the hood prior to preparation		
Inspected all products for particulate matter/contamination prior to use		
Cleared ampule neck of fluid before breaking		
Cleaned ampule neck correctly before breaking		
Wrapped ampule neck correctly before breaking		
Broke ampule correctly		
Attached filter device to syringe correctly		
Drew up ampule correctly, without spilling contents		
Removed filter needle and replaced it with new needle prior to injecting into final container		
Drew up the correct amount of drug and checked measurement prior to injecting into container		
Cleaned additive port on final container prior to injecting drug		
Did not core or puncture side of additive port when adding drug to the final container		
Properly mixed contents of container and inspected for incompatibilities or particulate matter		
Placed IV container in a zip-lock bag before removal from the hood		
Used any and all appropriate hazardous labeling (for product and waste)		
Properly sealed additive port of container		
Did not contaminate the needle or syringe during preparation		
Did not contaminate the hood		
Did not block airflow from HEPA filter or air intake grills at any time		
Did not utilize outer 6 in. of the hood opening		
Properly discarded all waste, including sharps		

By signing below, I certify that the student has demonstrated 100% competency at the above task.

____
Trainer Name (printed)

____
Trainer Signature

______________________________ ______________________________
Trainer Daytime Phone Trainer's License #

______________________________ ______________________________
Date State Licensed

Figure C-18

Process Validation Record

Vial Preparation—Hazardous Drugs

Student Name: ______________________ Date: __________

PROCEDURE	Yes	No
Followed proper hand-washing procedure and technique		
Wore appropriate apparel		
Followed proper procedure and technique in cleaning the hood		
Knew location of spill kit		
Knew location of eye wash station		
Performed all necessary calculations correctly prior to drug preparation		
Placed prep-mat/paper drape correctly prior to drug preparation		
Brought the correct drugs and concentrations into the hood for preparation		
Brought the correct supplies into the hood prior to preparation		
Inspected all products for particulate matter/contamination prior to use		
Removed dust covers and cleaned rubber diaphragms correctly		
Inserted needle correctly to prevent coring		
Used proper milking technique or venting device and didn't aspirate at any time		
Did not remove needle from vial until all air bubbles were removed and amount verified		
Removed air bubbles correctly and did not spill any liquid		
Withdrew needle correctly from vial to prevent spilling or aspiration		
Cleaned additive port on final container prior to injecting drug		
Did not core or puncture side of additive port when adding drug to the final container		
Properly mixed contents of container and inspected for incompatibilities or particulate matter		
Properly sealed additive port of container		
Placed IV container in a zip-lock bag before removal from the hood		
Used any and all appropriate hazardous labeling (for product and waste)		
Did not contaminate the needle or syringe during preparation		
Did not contaminate the hood		
Did not block airflow from HEPA filter or air intake grills at any time		
Did not utilize outer 6 in. of the hood opening		
Properly discarded all waste, including sharps		

By signing below, I certify that the student has demonstrated 100% competency at the above task.

____
Trainer Name (printed)

____
Trainer Signature

____
Trainer Daytime Phone

____
Trainer's License #

____
Date

____
State Licensed

Figure C-19

Process Validation Record

Sterile Ophthalmic Solution Preparation

Student Name: ______________________ Date: __________

PROCEDURE	Yes	No
Used horizontal airflow hood or other form of Class 100 sterile environment		
All containers, closures, droppers, and equipment were sterile		
Selected appropriate container and closure		
Selected appropriate preservative/buffer if needed		
Used appropriate filtration device		
Used proper aseptic technique		
Properly closed and sealed product before removal		
Used appropriate autoclave procedures if needed		
Did not remove hands from hood at any time during preparation		
Brought correct supplies and equipment to the hood		
Did not block the HEPA filter		
Placed appropriate labels on the final product		
Product was stored appropriately, or dispensed immediately		

By signing below, I certify that the student has demonstrated 100% competency at the above task.

Trainer Name (printed)

Trainer Signature

Trainer Daytime Phone

Trainer's License #

Date

State Licensed

Figure C-20

Process Validation Record

Sterile Product Label Preparation

Student Name: ______________________ Date: __________

PROCEDURE	**Yes**	**No**
Label followed the appropriate format, approved by the institution		
Label contained the name and amount of all solutions		
Label contained the name and amount of all additives		
Label contained name and identification/room number of the patient		
Label contained rate of administration, if applicable		
Label contained proper storage information		
Label contained date and time for administration		
Label contained an expiration date		
Label contained identification of the preparer and pharmacist in charge		
Label was properly affixed		
Label did not contain any errors or corrections		
Performed appropriate calculations as required to prepare the label		
Accurately transcribed information on the label from the physician's order		

By signing below, I certify that the student has demonstrated 100% competency at the above task.

____
Trainer Name (printed)

____
Trainer Signature

____
Trainer Daytime Phone

____
Trainer's License #

____
Date

____
State Licensed

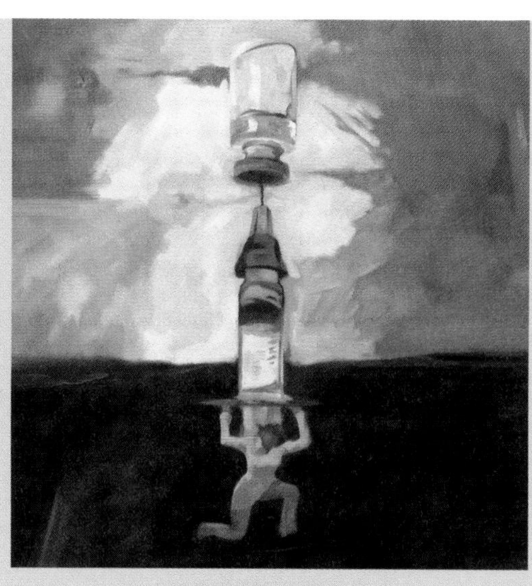

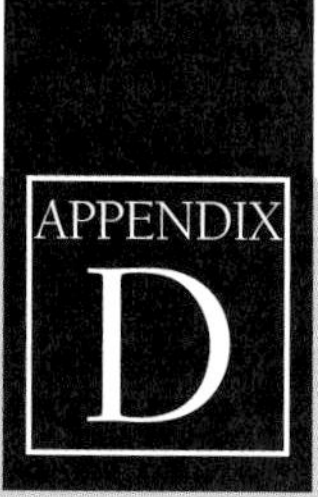

APPENDIX D

Instructions for Left-Handed Personnel

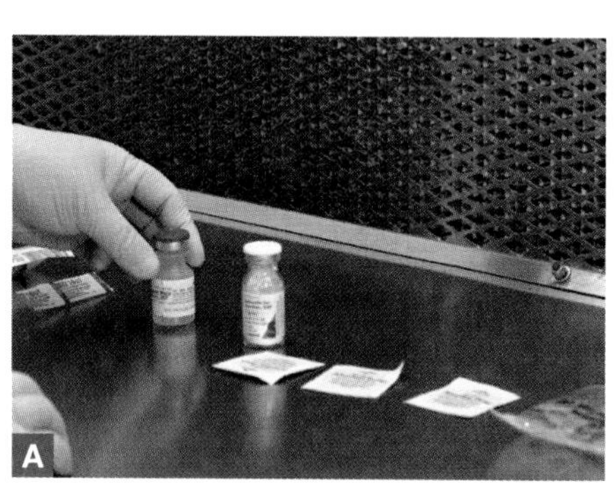

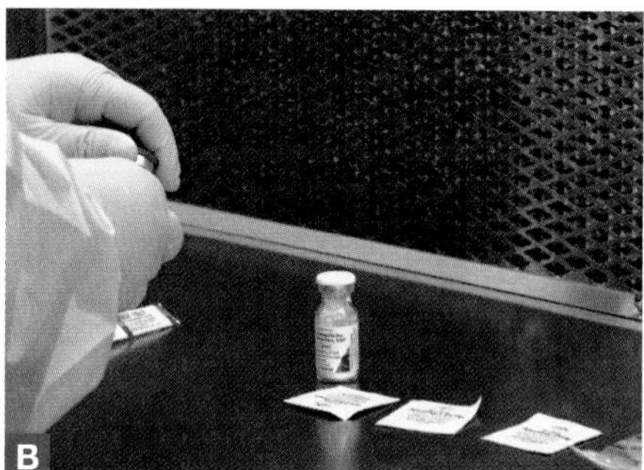

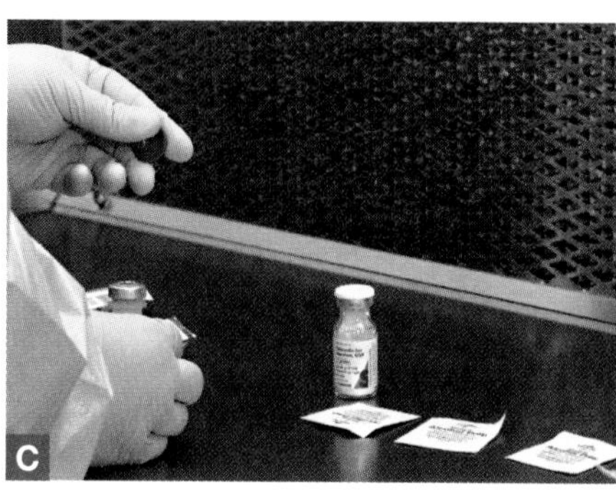

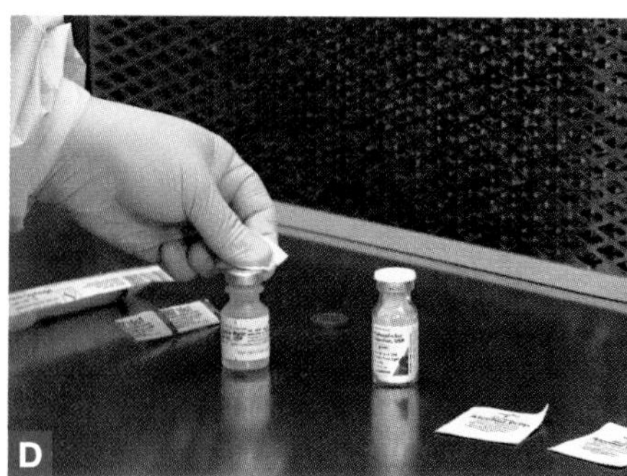

Figure D-1 Opening a vial (left hand)

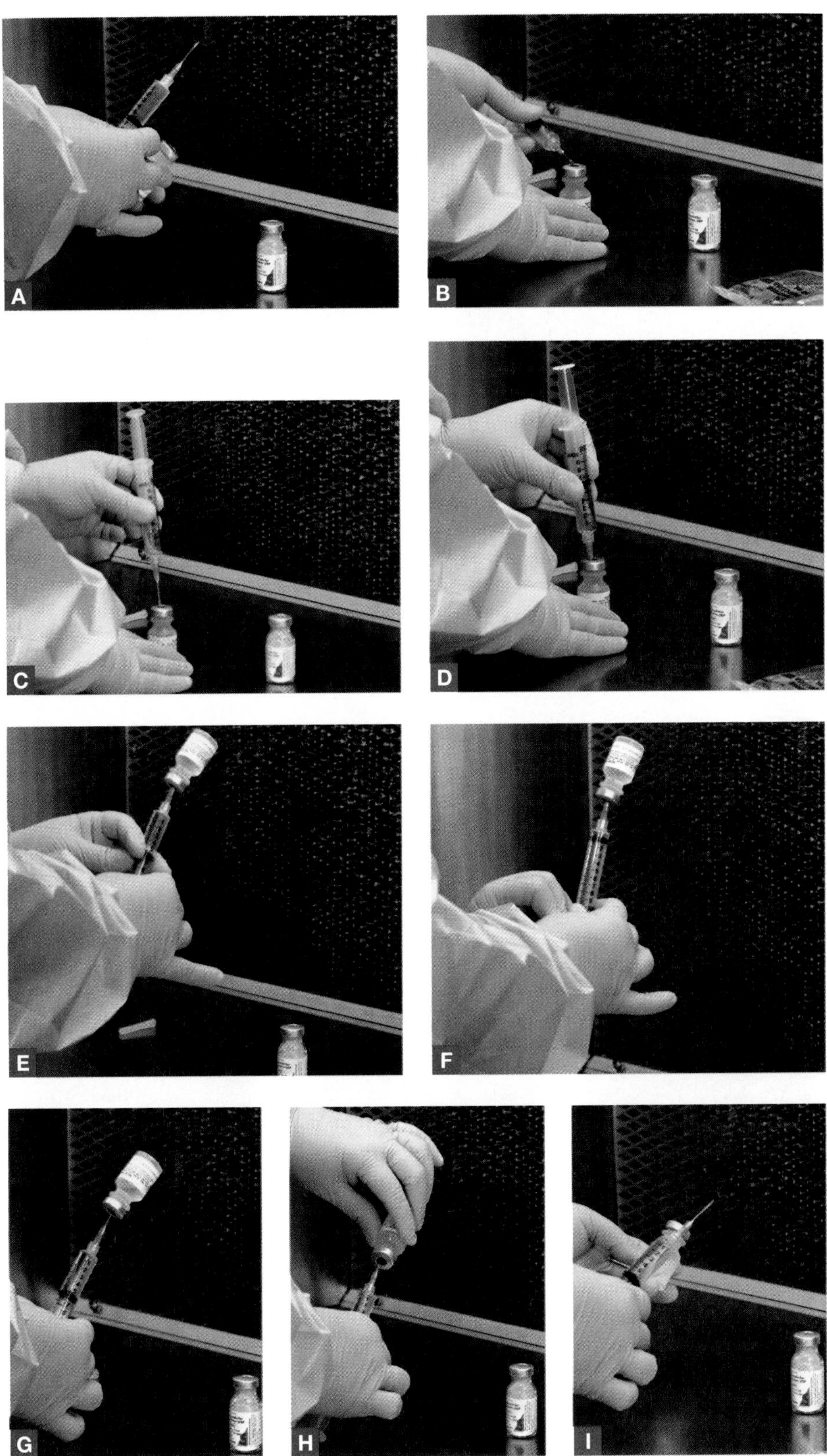

Figure D-2 Straight draw (left hand)

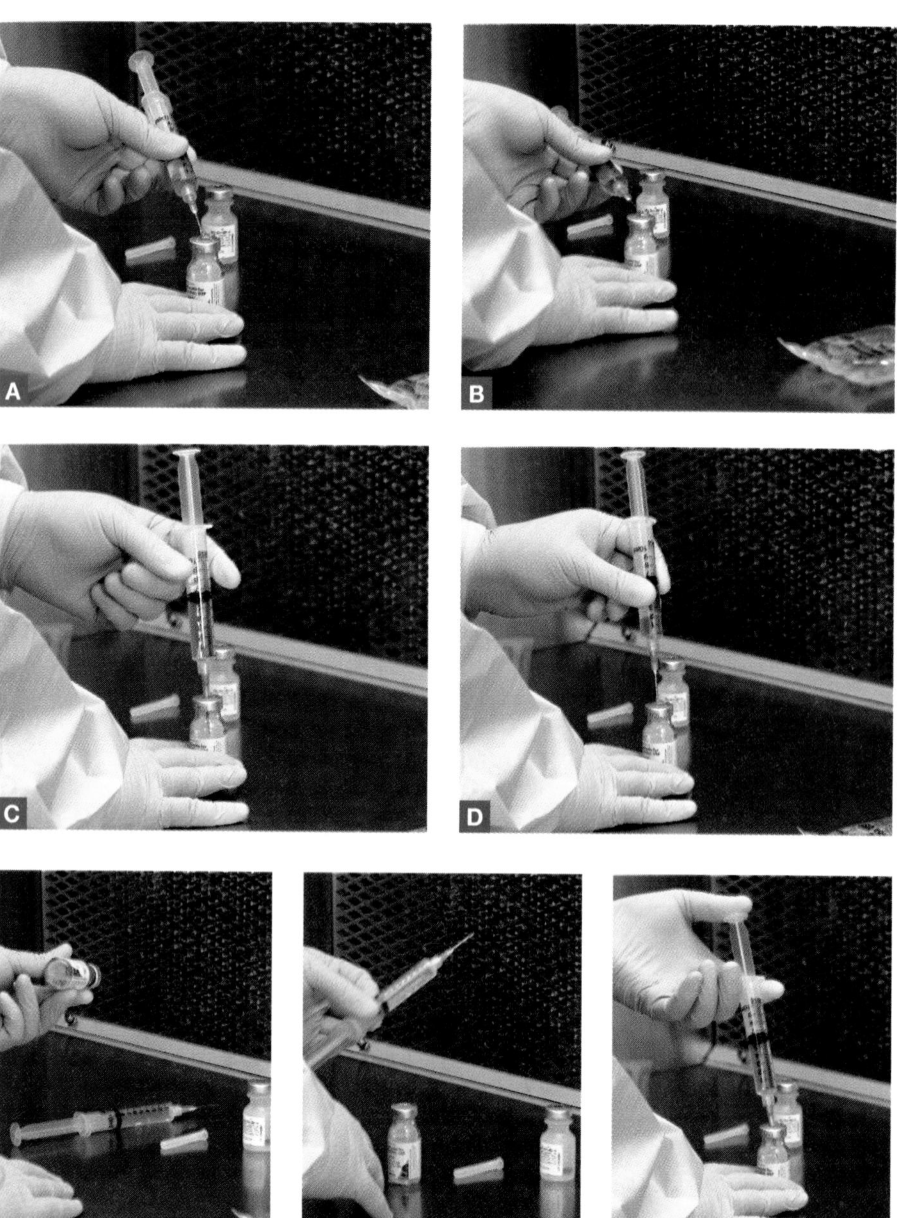

Figure D-3
Reconstitution of a lyophilized powder (left hand)

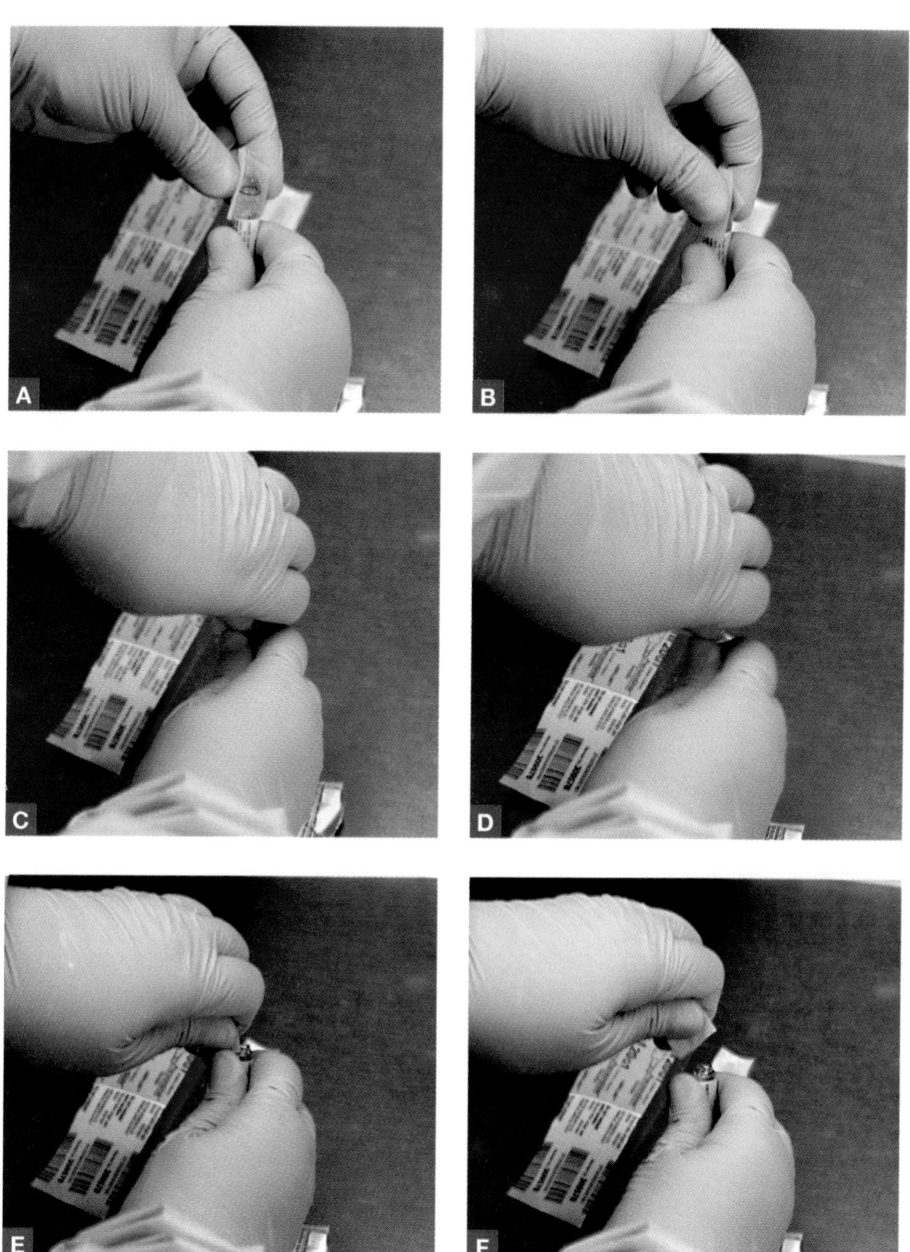

Figure D-4
Opening/breaking an ampule (left hand)

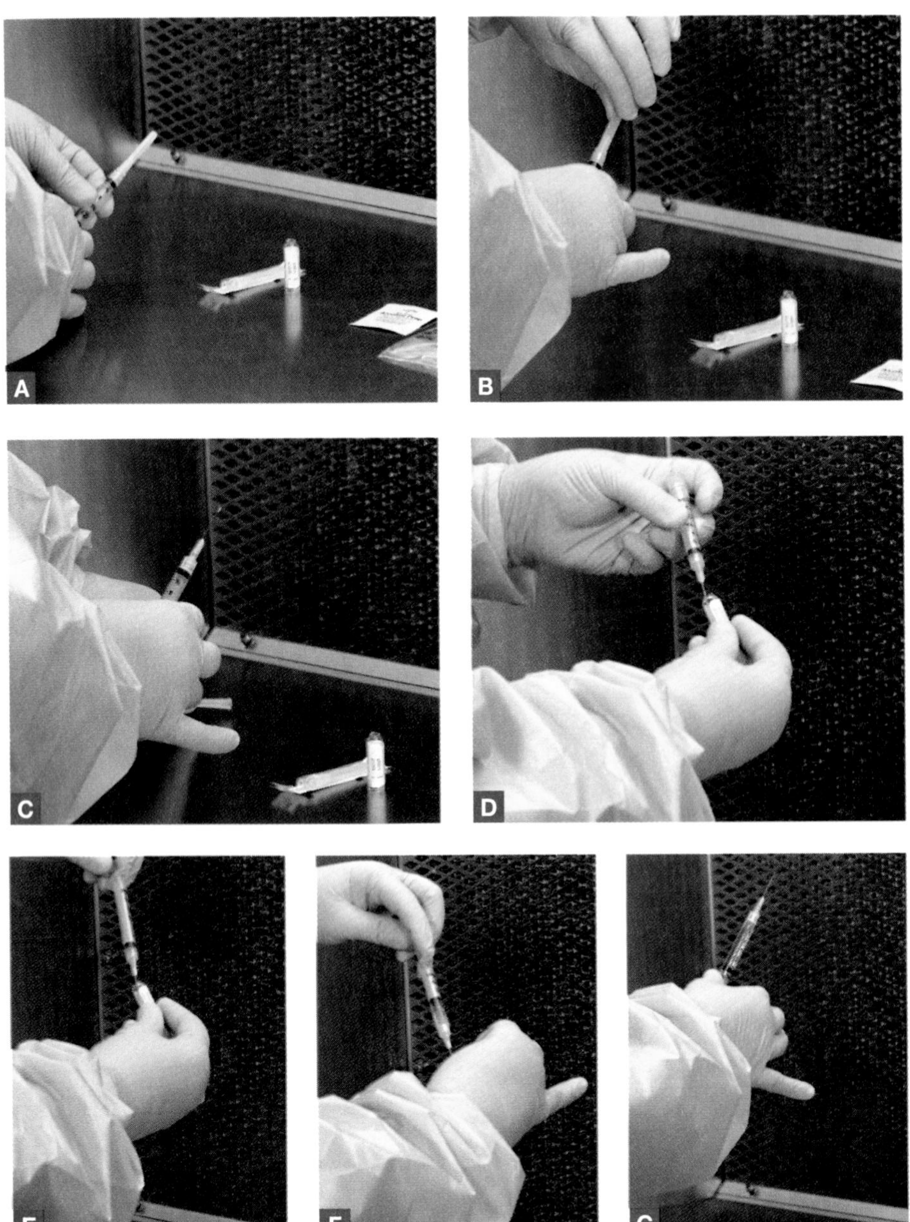

Figure D-5 Withdrawing fluid from an ampule (left hand)

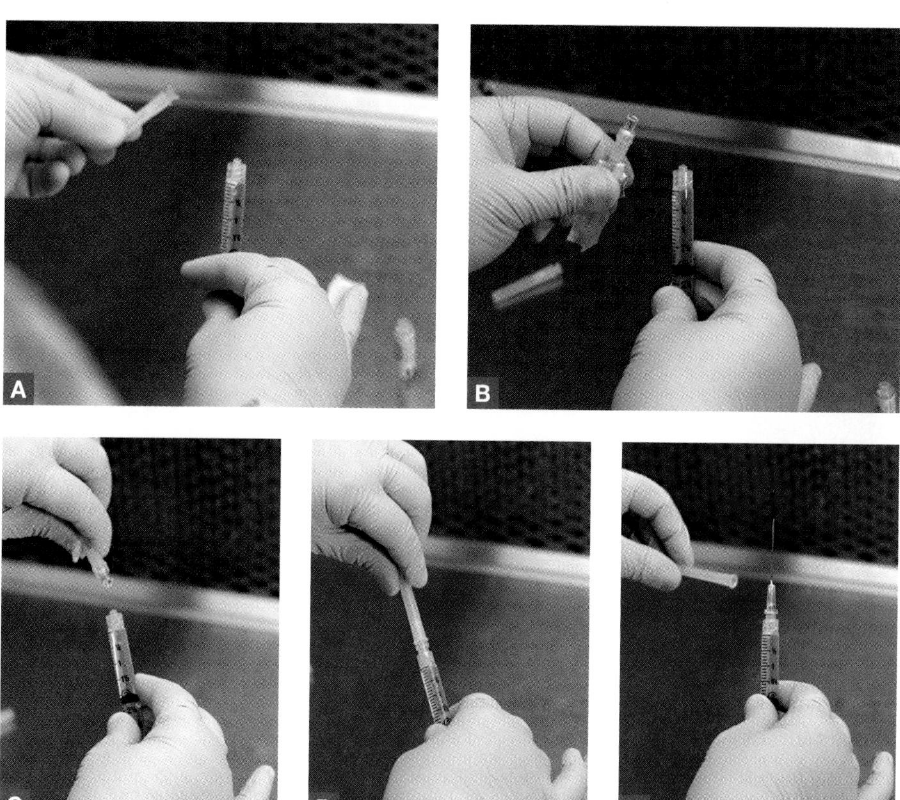

Figure D-6 Changing a needle (left hand)

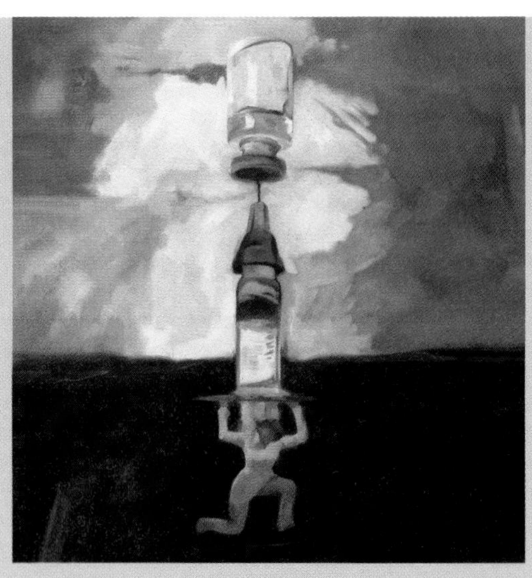

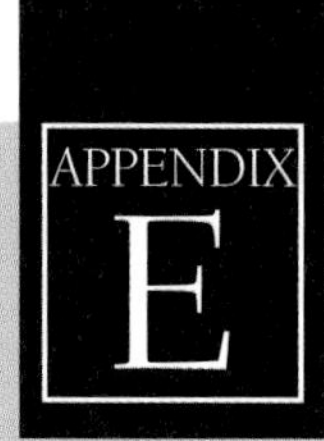

Resources and References

1. American Society of Health-System Pharmacists. "ASHP Guidelines on Quality Assurance for Pharmacy-Prepared Sterile Products," *American Journal of Health-System Pharmacists* 57 (2000): 1150–1169. (Also online at **www.ashp.org/bestpractices/drugdistribution/Prep_Gdl_QualAssur Sterile.pdf**.)
2. ———. *Manual for Pharmacy Technicians*. Bethesda, Md.: ASHP, 1998.
3. ———. "Technical Assistance Bulletin on Quality Assurance for Pharmacy-Prepared Sterile Products." Bethesda, Md.: ASHP, 1993.
4. American Society of Health-System Pharmacists Home Page. March 2005. **http://www.ashp.org**.
5. The Anaesthesia Education Website. "Fluid Physiology: 2.3 Osmolality and Tonicity." January 2005. **http://www.qldanaesthesia.com/FluidBook/FL2–3.htm**.
6. Ballington, Don. *Pharmacy Practice for Technicians*, 2nd ed. St. Paul, Minn.: EMC Paradigm, 2003.
7. Bradshaw, M. C., Garcia, D. E., and Wilroy, L. J. *Pharmacy Sterile Products Training Manual*. Houston, Texas: Pharmacy Education Resources, 1999.
8. Buchanan, E. Clyde. *Principles of Sterile Product Preparation*, rev. ed. Bethesda, Md.: American Society of Health-System Pharmacists, 1995.
9. Centers for Disease Control and Prevention. **http://www.cdc.gov**.
10. Drugs.com Home Page. March 2005. **http://www.drugs.com**.
11. Durgin, Jane M., and Hanan, Zachary I. *Pharmacy Practice for Technicians*, 3rd ed. Clifton Park, N.Y.: Delmar, 2005.
12. Drug Facts and Comparisons, 58th ed. St. Louis, MO: Wolters Kluwer Health, 2004.

13. Hunt, Max L., Jr. *Training Manual for Intravenous Admixture Personnel*, 5th ed. Lexington, Ky.: Precept Press, 1995.
14. Joint Commission on Accreditation of Healthcare Organizations Home Page. March 2005. **http://www.jcaho.org**.
15. National Home Infusion Association Home Page. March 2005. **http://www.nhianet.org**.
16. National Institute of Environmental Health Sciences. "Table 2: Comparison of Biosafety Cabinet Characteristics." January 2001. **http://www.niehs.nih.gov/odhsb/biosafe/bsc/table2.htm**.
17. PharmCatalyst Home Page. March 2005. **http://www.pharmcatalyst.com**.
18. RxKinetics Home Page. March 2005. **http://www.rxkinetics.com**.
19. Schafermeyer, Kenneth W. *The Pharmacy Technician Training Program*. 2003.
20. Shrewsbury, Robert. *Applied Pharmaceutics in Contemporary Compounding*. Englewood, Colo.: Morton, 2001.
21. Stoogenke, Marvin M. *The Pharmacy Technician*, 3rd ed. Upper Saddle River, N.J.: Prentice Hall, 2001.
22. United States Pharmacopeia. "Pharmaceutical Compounding: Sterile Preparations" (USP Chapter 797). Rockville, Md.: USP, 2004.
23. United States Pharmacopeia. "Sterile Drug Products for Home Use" (USP Chapter 1206). Rockville, Md.: USP, 1995.
24. U.S. Food and Drug Administration Home Page. March 2005. **http://www.fda.gov**.
25. Wilroy, Liz Johnson, and Garcia, Daniel E. *Pharmacy Sterile Products Training Manual*. Houston, Texas: Pharmacy Education Resources, 2002.

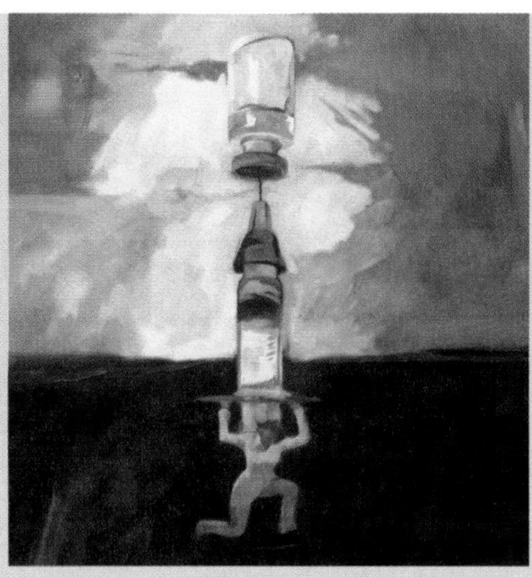

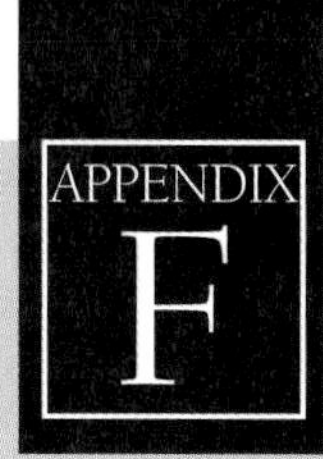

Answers

Chapter 1
Introduction to Sterile Products

ANSWERS TO CHAPTER REVIEW QUESTIONS

1. a. inhalants
2. c. topicals
3. e. parenterals
4. f. oral
5. e. parenterals
6. f. oral
7. e. parenterals
8. e. parenterals
9. e. parenterals
10. d. ophthalmics and otics
11. e. a, b, and c
12. g. medication or fluid administered into the dermis
13. f. medication or fluid administered under the dermis
14. a. medication or fluid administered into the muscle
15. d. medication administered into the cardiac muscle
16. b. medication or fluid administered into the epidural space, which is the outer layer of the spinal cord
17. e. medication or fluid administered into the subarachnoid space surrounding the spinal cord
18. c. medication or fluid administered into a vein
19. a.
20. a.
21. a.
22. a.
23. b.
24. b.
25. a.

Chapter 2
Facilities, Garb, and Equipment

ANSWERS TO CHAPTER REVIEW QUESTIONS

1. c. cardboard boxes
2. c. paper towels
3. e. a, b, and c
4. a. sterile water, 70% isopropyl alcohol, lint-free paper towels/gauze
5. c. vertical from top to bottom
6. b. glass shards and other particulates from a solution
7. c. leur-to-leur connectors
8. b. Dispensing pins
9. a. Viaflex bags
10. a. 30 min
11. c. monthly

Chapter 3
Aseptic Calculations

PRACTICE PROBLEMS 3.1

1. 1 g
2. 1 g
3. 0.120 g
4. 7.5 mL
5. 20 min
6. 6 mL
7. 83 gtt./min
8. 200 gtt./min
9. a. 6 mL b. 6 mL c. 6 mL
   d. 10 mL e. 5 mL f. 19 mL
   g. 5 mL h. 38.7 mL i. 95.7 mL
10. four dilutions

ANSWERS TO CHAPTER REVIEW QUESTIONS

1. c. 72.73 kg
2. a. 18,182,500 U/day
3. c. 91 mL, 909 mL
4. c. 38 mL/hr
5. c. 12,602 U/min
6. b. 20 kg
7. d. 5.0 mg
8. a. 0.015 g
9. c. 1.25 mL
10. d. 33 gtt./min

Chapter 4
Properties of Sterile Products

ANSWERS TO CHAPTER REVIEW QUESTIONS

1. d. hypertonic
2. d. hypotonic
3. d. both b and c
4. b. 7.4
5. a. physical, chemical, therapeutic
6. e. none of the above
7. b. The pH balance is not equal between the eyes and the soap.
8. e. 24–48 hr
9. b. 0
10. a. isotonic

CHAPTER 5

Aseptic Technique

ANSWERS TO CHAPTER REVIEW QUESTIONS

1. a. anteroom
2. c. PPE
3. d. 6 in.
4. a. 30 min
5. e. glass
6. c. reconstitution
7. b. filters
8. a. 20 percent
9. d. the alcohol to dry completely
10. b. date them
11. d. to prevent foaming

CHAPTER 6

Sterile Product Preparations

ANSWERS TO CHAPTER REVIEW QUESTIONS

1. b. IV bags
2. c. intravenous piggybacks
3. d. send up the bottle and the nurse can draw up the test
4. b. IVPB
5. c. large volume
6. b. The IV technician should never put narcotics in an epidural.
7. c. Advantage
8. e. personal controlled anesthesia
9. a. irrigation
10. e. 30 min

CHAPTER 7

Total Parenteral Nutrition (TPN)

ANSWERS TO CHAPTER REVIEW QUESTIONS

1. c. total parenteral nutrition
2. a. the food bag
3. d. potassium phosphate and calcium gluconate
4. d. physicians
5. b. pharmacists
6. e. all of the above
7. b. in a laminar airflow hood
8. d. multivitamin for injection

MATCHING

9. a
10. b
11. b
12. b
13. a
14. b
15. b
16. a
17. b
18. b
19. b
20. a
21. b
22. b
23. b
24. b
25. a
26. b
27. b
28. b
29. a
30. b

CHAPTER 8
Chemotherapy

ANSWERS TO CHAPTER REVIEW QUESTIONS

1. e. all of the above
2. c. fast-growing cells
3. e. all of the above
4. c. from the top of the hood
5. a. yellow hazardous disposal container
6. c. They must be washed.
7. d. physician
8. b. pharmacist
9. c. six months
10. a. a sealable zip-lock container
11. d. 5 mL

CHAPTER 9
Quality Control and Assurance

ANSWERS TO CHAPTER REVIEW QUESTIONS

1. b. the five rights
2. c. microbial contamination
3. d. Joint Commission on Accreditation of Healthcare Organizations
4. e. USP 797
5. d. competency, training, education
6. b. end product evaluation
7. b. 100
8. d. 2° to 8° C
9. a. quality
10. a. United States Pharmacopeia

Index

C

N

O

P

Q

R

S

T

U

V

W

Y